CASE STUDIES

IN

CLINICAL

PHARMACOLOGY

Case Studies in Clinical Pharmacology

Grant, Marcia Moeller, R.N., M.S.N., Research Associate, Department of Nursing Research, City of Hope National Medical Center, Duarte, California

McFarland, Mary Brambilla, R.N., M.S.N., Assistant Professor, School of Nursing, University of Oregon, Portland, Oregon

Kubo, Winifred Matsui, R.N., M.S.N., Assistant Professor, Department of Professional Nursing, School of Nursing, University of Hawaii, Honolulu, Hawaii

Weatherford, Rosalie Wooding, R.N., M.S.N., Assistant Professor, Department of Nursing, J. Sargeant Reynolds Community College, Richmond, Virginia

Ehlke, Graceann, R.N., M.S.N., Instructor, School of Nursing, University of Hawaii, Honolulu, Hawaii

F. A. DAVIS COMPANY

PHILADELPHIA

Library of Congress Cataloging Card Number 77-73676

ISBN 0-8036-3080-8

PREFACE

The case studies in this book have been designed to assist the nurse with the integration and application of pharmacology in the clinical nursing care of adult medicosurgical patients. Patient situations that reflect common and major adult health problems are used as a means of linking theoretical knowledge regarding drug actions to the application of appropriate nursing care. This is accomplished by

1. Relating drug action to specific pathophysiological processes.

2. Defining areas for nursing assessment regarding therapeutic, side and toxic effects.

3. Defining specific nursing actions to enhance therapeutic effects and to prevent and minimize side and toxic effects.

References include current clinical nursing and pharmacology textbooks as well as current articles from a variety of periodicals.

CONTENTS

ABBREVIATIONS

a.c.	before meals
b.i.d.	twice a day
BUN	blood urea nitrogen
cm	centimeter
CPK	creatinine phosphokinase
CVP	central venous pressure
EKG	electrocardiogram
F.	Fahrenheit
gm	gram
Hg	mercury
hr.	hour
h.s.	hour of sleep
IM	intramuscular
IPPB	intermittent positive pressure breathing
IV	intravenous
kg	kilogram
LDH	lactic dehydrogenase
mEq	milliequivalent
mEq/L	milliequivalent per liter
mg	milligram
ml	milliliter
mm	millimeter
mOs	milliosmols
NPO	nothing by mouth
$PaCO_2$	arterial carbon dioxide tension
PaO_2	arterial oxygen tension
p.c.	after meals
pH	power of the hydrogen ion
p.o.	by mouth
PPD	purified protein derivative
p.r.n.	whenever necessary
PVC	premature ventricular contractions
q.i.d.	four times a day
s.c.	subcutaneous
SGOT	serum glutamic oxaloacetic transaminase
SGPT	serum glutamic pyruvic transaminase
stat.	as soon as possible
tabs	tablets
t.i.d.	three times a day
U	units
VDRL	venereal disease research laboratories

1

THE PATIENT WITH GLAUCOMA

TEXTBOOKS SUGGESTED FOR THIS STUDY

Bergersen, G.: Pharmacology in Nursing, ed. 13. C. V. Mosby Co., St.Louis, 1976, Chapter 29.
Brunner, L. S., and Suddarth, D.: Textbook of Medical Surgical Nursing, ed. 3. J. B. Lippincott Co., Philadelphia, 1975, Chapter 33.
Goodman, L., and Gilman, A. (eds.): The Pharmacological Basis of Therapeutics, ed. 5. Macmillan Co., New York, 1975, Chapters 22 and 23.
Luckmann, J., and Sorensen, K.: Medical-Surgical Nursing — A Psychophysiologic Approach. W. B. Saunders Co., Philadelphia, 1974, Chapter 105.
Rodman, M. J., and Smith, D.: Clinical Pharmacology in Nursing. J. B. Lippincott Co., Philadelphia, 1974, Chapters 21 and 22.
Shafer, K. N., et al.: Medical Surgical Nursing, ed. 6. C. V. Mosby Co., St. Louis, 1975, Chapter 31.

PAST MEDICAL HISTORY

Thelma Green was a 65-year-old widow who had been in good physical health. Her medical history was essentially negative for cardiovascular, respiratory, and renal diseases. There was no history of diabetes, surgery, or allergies to food or drugs. There were no significant findings on the physical examination.

First Office Visit (Saturday)

Mrs. Green was referred to an ophthalmologist by her internist because of complaints of blurred vision, headaches, dull eye pain, and seeing halos around objects for the past few months.

Her vital signs were temperature 98.6° F., pulse 72, respirations 18, and blood pressure 130/80. Her intraocular pressure was elevated in both eyes. The pressure was measured in her left eye at 40 mm Hg and in her right eye at 35 mm Hg. After a thorough examination she was diagnosed as having chronic glaucoma (wide angle).

Medical Orders

(1) Isoflurophate (DFP) 1 drop in each eye daily
(2) Return visit on Monday

While interviewing Mrs. Green, the nurse obtained additional information. Mrs. Green, an alert and active woman, lived alone in a third-story flat since her husband's death 10 years before. She was a retired school teacher active in a Golden Age Club. She used to drive to various activities, picking up three or four other women who were also members of the club. She stated that she became frightened and quit driving when she nearly hit a car in the next lane while attempting to change lanes. She failed to see the car alongside until one of her passengers warned her. She expressed a desire to continue her activity with the club and stated she would take the bus. She particularly enjoyed the evening outings to plays, concerts, and bridge parties. She played tennis regularly since she was very young and enjoyed this form of exercise. She also did a great deal of reading when she was not occupied with her other activities. Her married daughter, with whom she was in touch daily, lived about 10 minutes away from her.

Study Questions

1. How does isoflurophate reduce Mrs. Green's intraocular pressure?

2. Relate the signs and symptoms of the side effects for isoflurophate to its pharmacologic action.

3. Mrs. Green has never instilled eye drops before. Describe important points which she must learn regarding self-administration of eye drops.

4. When is the best time for administration of isoflurophate? Why?

5. Ophthalmologic drugs include the following categories: cholinergic, anticholinergic, anticholinesterase, adrenergic, and carbonic anhydrase inhibitor drugs. To which category does isoflurophate belong? Compare adverse and side effects of drugs of each category when administered as eye drops. State indications for ophthalmologic drugs in each category.

6. Of what significance is the initial blood pressure record in isoflurophate administration?

7. What types of preexisting health problems would be contra-indications for the use of anticholinesterase drugs?

8. Mrs. Green asks how long she will need to have eye drops. Describe instructions to be given to her regarding length of administration of medication for her glaucoma.

Second Office Visit (Monday)

Mrs. Green's intraocular pressure was recorded as left eye 25 mm Hg and right eye 22 mm Hg. Mrs. Green related that she was dizzy, nauseated, and had episodes of diarrhea since her visit on Saturday. She reported that she was salivating more than usual. She stated that although her eye pain had subsided, her vision was still blurred and her headache seemed worse. Vital signs were temperature 98.8° F., pulse 90, respirations 20, and blood pressure 100/60.

Medical Orders

(1) Discontinue isoflurophate
(2) Pilocarpine 1% 1 drop in each eye t.i.d.
(3) Return visit tomorrow

Study Questions

9. Why was the order changed to pilocarpine? What is the action of pilocarpine?

10. What are the advantages and disadvantages of pilocarpine compared to isoflurophate?

11. What is the risk with long term administration of a potent anticholinesterase agent?

12. What evidence of drug effectiveness is present at this visit?

13. If Mrs. Green's symptoms progress to include a further drop in blood pressure and an asthmatic type attack, what antidote is usually prescribed?

Third Office Visit (Tuesday)

Intraocular pressure was recorded as left eye 28 mm Hg and right eye 25 mm Hg. Mrs. Green stated that she still had diarrhea and excessive salivation and her headache persisted. The nurse asked Mrs. Green to describe and demonstrate how she was instilling her eye drops. Mrs. Green reported feeling drops of medication leak down into her nose. She also mentioned that she will be hospitalized next month for a hysterectomy. She related that her daughter was encouraging her to move from her third-story flat to an apartment on the first floor, or into her daughter's home, which was on one floor. Mrs. Green stated, "My daughter seemed concerned about the three flights and the dark stairwell, I guess. But I don't want to move."

Medical Orders

(1) Pilocarpine 2% 1 drop in each eye t.i.d.
(2) Acetozolamide (Diamox) 250 mg t.i.d.

Study Questions

14. What is the reason from the description of the third office visit for the increase in pilocarpine dosage and the addition of acetozolamide?

15. How is acetozolamide administered? Describe the times at which Mrs. Green should be instructed to take both medications.

16. How does acetozolamide reduce intraocular pressure? Relate the side effects of acetozolamide to its pharmacological action.

17. What additional patient teaching is required now that Mrs. Green will also be

taking acetozolamide?

18. During this office visit, why was the nurse asking Mrs. Green about her method of eye drop instillation?

19. Based on the information from Mrs. Green, what teaching regarding eye drop instillation must be reinforced at this time?

20. In relation to Mrs. Green's impending surgery, what drug is routinely given preoperatively which will counteract the effect of pilocarpine? What other nursing actions are indicated to insure continuity of care for Mrs. Green's glaucoma during hospitalization for her hysterectomy?

21. It is essential to share what information about pilocarpine action with Mrs. Greene to help her understand the reality of her daughter's concern?

22. What kind of counseling is needed regarding Mrs. Green's varied activities which she described during her first office visit? (i.e. Will she be able to drive again? Can she continue to play tennis and read as in the past? Can she continue her evening outings?) Which drug is most apt to affect her leisure activities and why?

Fourth, Fifth, and Sixth Office Visits (Wednesday, Thursday, and Friday)

For the next three visits, Mrs. Green's intraocular pressure was recorded as left eye 20 mm Hg and right eye 18 mm Hg. She reported absence of the headache, no halos around objects, and decreased blurring of vision. However, there was no change in peripheral visual field defects. Mrs. Green stated that since her vision seemed to have improved so much she would like to drive again.

Medical Orders

(1) Continue same medications
(2) Return visit Monday

Study Questions

23. What evidence of drug effectiveness is present during these visits?

24. Regarding Mrs. Green's desire to resume driving, what counseling is needed?

Seventh Office Visit (Monday)

Pressures recorded remained within normal range. Mrs. Green complained that she was again nauseated and was also weak and tired. When questioned about her diet, Mrs. Green stated that she had put herself on a low-bulk diet with no fresh fruits or vegetables since her last bout with diarrhea. Laboratory tests were ordered immediately.

Laboratory Results

Serum sodium	130 mEq/L
Serum potassium	3.2 mEq/L

Medical Orders

(1) Discontinue acetozolamide (Diamox)
(2) Continue pilocarpine
(3) Resume well balanced diet
(4) Return in three days

Study Questions

25. How are Mrs. Green's complaints and resultant laboratory tests related to her glaucoma therapy?

26. How might this episode have been prevented?

27. What suggestions regarding immediate dietary intake are indicated?

28. What additional instruction is necessary regarding continuance of eye drops in the event that Mrs. Green is too ill to administer them herself?

Progress Report

Mrs. Green was seen weekly for two more weeks with continued normal intraocular pressures and absence of other complaints. She was scheduled for a return visit in three months.

Study Questions

29. What other modes of therapy are available to the patient with wide angle glaucoma if medications fail to effectively reduce intraocular pressure?

REFERENCES

Armaly, M.: Glaucoma. Arch. Ophthalmol., 90:485-501, 1973.
Condl, E. D.: Ophthalmic nursing: the gentle touch. Nurs. Clin. N. Am., 5:449-496, 1970.
Haddad, H. M.: Drugs for ophthalmic use. Am. J. Nurs., 68:324-327, 1968.
Modell, W. (Ed.): Drugs of Choice, 1976-1977. C. V. Mosby Co., St. Louis, 1976.
Seaman, F.: Nursing care of the glaucoma patient. Nurs. Clin. N. Am., 5:489-496, 1970.
Soll, D. B.: Glaucoma. Nurs. Digest, 3:9-12, 1975.
Shiery, S.: Insight into the delicate art of eye care. Nursing '75, 5:50-56, 1975.

2

THE PATIENT WITH CHRONIC CYSTITIS

TEXTBOOKS SUGGESTED FOR THIS STUDY

Asperheim, M. K., and Eisenhauer, L. A.: The Pharmacologic Basis of Patient Care. W. B. Saunders Co., Philadelphia, 1973, Chapter 9.
Bergerson, B.: Pharmacology in Nursing, ed. 13. C. V. Mosby Co., St. Louis, 1976, Chapters 19 and 20.
Brunner, L. S., and Suddarth, D. S.: Textbook of Medical-Surgical Nursing, ed. 3. J. B. Lippincott Co., Philadelphia, 1975, Chapter 26.
Goodman, L., and Gilman, A. (eds.): The Pharmacological Basis of Therapeutics, ed. 5. Macmillan Co., New York, 1975, Chapters 50, 56, and 57.
Luckmann, J., and Sorensen, K.: Medical-Surgical Nursing — A Psychophysiologic Approach. W. B. Saunders Co., Philadelphia, 1974, Chapter 57.
Rodman, M. J., and Smith, D. W.: Pharmacology and Drug Therapy in Nursing. J. B. Lippincott Co., Philadelphia, 1974, Chapters 40, 41, and 42.
Shafer, K., et al.: Medical-Surgical Nursing, ed. 6. C. V. Mosby Co., St. Louis, 1975, Chapter 20.

First Clinic Visit

Mary Gonzales, a 24-year-old woman, visited the outpatient clinic shortly after her marriage complaining of burning, urgent, and frequent urination. A urine culture showed over 100,00 colonies of Escherichia coli and the diagnosis of acute "honeymoon" cystitis was made. The physician prescribed sulfisoxazole 0.5 gm with phenazopyridine hydrochloride 50 mg (Azogantrisin) 4 tablets stat. and 1 tablet q.i.d. for 10 days. Within 48 hours the symptoms subsided and a repeat midstream urine culture a week later showed a marked decrease in bacteriuria. The nurse instructed Mrs. Gonzales to return to the clinic for a urine culture if she ever had the same symptoms again.

Fifth Clinic Visit (Four Months Later)

Mrs. Gonzales returned with bladder infections each month. These infections were accompanied by local symptoms of dysuria, urgency, and frequency and her urine cultures showed several colonies of Escherichia coli. She did not notice any fatigue or fever with these episodes. Mrs. Gonzales was treated successfully on three occasions with Azogantrisin; however, for her current infection, she was given ampicillin (Polycillin) 50 mg p.o. to be taken every 6 hours for 10 days, and phenazopyridine (Pyridium) 100 mg p.o. t.i.d. for 4 days. Before leaving the clinic, Mrs. Gonzales talked to the nurse about her frequent infections and expressed concern about having to take the new medicine every six hours saying that it probably didn't matter when she took it.

Study Questions

1. Azogantrisin contains sulfisoxazole and phenazopyridine. Describe the pharmacologic action of each of these medications and the site at which that action occurs.

2. What are the therapeutic effects that occur following treatment with Azogantrisin? Consider the signs and symptoms exhibited by Mrs. Gonzales in your answer.

3. Serious toxic effects may occur with the administration of any medication containing sulfisoxazole. What are these effects? How can the nurse instruct Mrs. Gonzales so that she might avoid these toxic effects?

4. What should the nurse tell Mrs. Gonzales about the phenazopyridine component of Azogantrisin?

5. Why was Mrs. Gonzales' medication changed to ampicillin after she had several courses of treatment with Azogantrisin?

6. Ampicillin is a synthetic penicillin. Compare its bacterial activity and pharmacologic actions to those of penicillin.

7. For what types of infections is ampicillin most effective? Why was it ordered every 6 hours instead of four times a day?

8. Discuss the problems of patient compliance to medication therapy on an outpatient basis when a drug is ordered every 6 hours versus twice a day. What suggestions might the nurse make to increase patient compliance?

9. What important nursing measures must be taken before and after a patient is given a medication containing the properties of penicillin? Include the responsibilities of both the hospital and clinic nurse when giving your answer.

10. How should the nurse explain the reason for the change of medication to Mrs. Gonzales?

11. Describe how a plan for taking the medicine on time could be developed with this patient.

Seventh Clinic Visit (Six Months Later)

Mrs. Gonzales had recurrent infections whenever the administration of ampicillin was discontinued. On this clinic visit her cystitis was treated with sulfisoxazole (Gantrisin) 0.5 mg p.o. q.i.d. which she was instructed to take for 3 months.

Eighth Clinic Visit (One Year Later)

On her next clinic visit, Mrs. Gonzales' midstream urine culture was negative for bacteria and she reported no other urinary symptoms. Her sulfisoxazole was decreased to 0.5 mg p.o. to be taken before and after sexual intercourse. Mrs. Gonzales asked the clinic nurse to explain the reason she had to take her medicine in this manner and also asked if this would affect her ability to conceive a child.

Eleventh Clinic Visit (One Year Later)

Mrs. Gonzales said that she did not have any signs or symptoms of infection during the three months prior to this clinic visit; however, she did say that she often had to get up in the middle of the night to urinate. A urine culture showed contamination with Escherichia coli and the physician recommended a complete urological workup. Mrs. Gonzales began to express concern to the clinic nurse about her medical care and wondered if the physician who was treating her really knew what was wrong, since none of the medications prevented her infections.

Study Questions

12. Why was sulfisoxazole ordered before and after sexual intercourse? How should the nurse tell Mrs. Gonzales to take this medication?

13. What would have been an appropriate response to Mrs. Gonzales when she asked if she would be able to conceive a child?

14. Mrs. Gonzales expressed concern about her medical care and the unsuccessful attempt to prevent her urinary tract infections. How could the nurse explain the reasons for her continued infection and the different medications she has received? Consider the chronic nature of cystitis in your answer.

Laboratory Results

Mrs. Gonzales' excretory urogram (intravenous pyelogram) and retrograde cystogram were negative. Her cystoscopy revealed a pseudomembrane in the area of the trigone of her bladder.

Medical Orders

Sulfamethoxazole (Gantanol) 1.0 gm b.i.d. for 3 months

Thirteenth Clinic Visit (One Year and Four Months Later)

Two weeks after she completed taking the 3-month supply of sulfamethoxazole (Gantanol), Mrs. Gonzales had recurrent lower urinary tract symptoms of urgency, burning, and frequency of urination. A urine culture again showed Escherichia coli. Nitrofurantoin macrocrystals (Macrodantin) 100 mg q.i.d. was ordered. After 10 days of medication therapy the dosage was reduced to nitrofurantoin macrocrystals 50 mg b.i.d. for 6 months.

Nineteenth Clinic Visit (One Year and Ten Months Later)

Urine cultures taken at one-month intervals were negative. Mrs. Gonzales was given nitrofurantoin macrocrystals 50 mg to take before and following coitus. She was pleased that she had been free from infection for so long and was reluctant to have her medication reduced.

Twentieth Clinic Visit (Two Years Later)

Mrs. Gonzales began to have urinary urgency and a urine culture showed Proteus mirabilis. Sulfamethoxazole 1.0 gm was prescribed to be taken b.i.d. for 4 months. Monthly urine cultures showed that she was free from infection and, after her course of sulfamethoxazole, she was placed on nitrofurantoin macrocrystals 100 mg every night. Mrs. Gonzales again felt reluctant to have her medication reduced; however, after a discussion with the clinic nurse about her concerns, she agreed to follow the prescribed medical regimen.

Study Questions

15. Compare the pharmacologic action and the frequency of adminsitration of sulfamethoxazole to sulfisoxazole.

16. Mrs. Gonzales' medication was changed several times during the course of her medical treatment. What should the nurse tell her about the reason for these changes? Relate these changes to the nature of chronic cystitis and the organisms involved.

17. Why was nitrofurantoin macrocrystals ordered instead of sulfamethoxazole when Mrs Gonzales had a recurrent infection? What should the nurse tell her about this change in medication?

18. Compare the action of nitrofurantoin macrocrystals to nitrofurantoin. What should the nurse tell patients about these medication when they are to be taken at home?

19. Compare the site of action of the sulfonamide medications to nitrofurantoin drugs.

20. During the course of her medical treatment, Mrs. Gonzales' infections would occur when her medication was reduced. What should the nurse tell her to help her understand the reasons for the medication reduction and the importance of her following the doctor's orders?

Progress Report

Frequent urine cultures showed that Mrs. Gonzales remained free from infection for two years. During that time she continued to take nitrofurantoin macrocrystals 100 mg every night. She became pregnant and remained free of urinary tract infections during the pregnancy. She took nitrofurantoin macrocrystals as prescribed except during the last six weeks of her pregnancy. Following the birth of her baby, Mrs. Gonzales was not given any medication and had no further problems with cystitis. Plans were made for evaluation of her progress in the Urology Clinic.

Study Questions

21. Discuss the ways in which medications taken during pregnancy may affect the growing fetus.

22. Why was Mrs. Gonzales' medication discontinued six weeks prior to her delivery date?

23. Although Mrs. Gonzales has been free of infection, what should the nurse tell her about the importance of follow-up care?

REFERENCES

Bailey, R. R., Roberts, A. P., Gower, P. E., and Wardener, H. E.: Prevention of urinary tract infections with low-dose nitrofurantoin. Lancet 2:1112-1114, 1971.

Kunin, N.: New developments in the diagnosis and treatment of urinary tract infections. J. Urol. 113:585-594, 1975.

Rodman, M. J.: Fighting the second most frequent infections, Part 1. R.N. 38:75-78, 1975.

Rodman, M. J.: Fighting the second most frequent infections, Part 2. R.N. 38:91-95, 1975.

3

THE PATIENT WITH A PEPTIC ULCER

TEXTBOOKS SUGGESTED FOR THIS STUDY

Asperheim, M. K., and Eisenhauer, L. A.: The Pharmacologic Basis of Patient Care. W. B. Saunders Co., Philadelphia, 1973, Chapters 6, 11, 12, and 17.

Bergersen, B.: Pharmacology in Nursing, ed. 13. C. V. Mosby Co., St. Louis, 1976, Chapters 9, 10, 11, 20, and 31.

Brunner, L. S., and Suddarth, D.: Textbook of Medical Surgical Nursing, ed. 3. J. B. Lippincott Co., Philadelphia, 1975, Chapter 24.

Goodman, L., and Gilman, A. (eds.): The Pharmacological Basis of Therapeutics, ed. 5. Macmillan Co., New York, 1975, Chapters 25, 48, and 63.

Luckmann, J., and Sorensen, K.: Medical-Surgical Nursing — A Psychophysiologic Approach. W. B. Saunders Co., Philadelphia, 1974, Chapter 78.

Rodman, M. J., and Smith, D.: Pharmacology and Drug Therapy in Nursing. J. B. Lippincott Co., Philadelphia, 1974, Chapters 13, 22, 34, and 41.

Shafer, K. N., et al.: Medical Surgical Nursing, ed. 6. C. V. Mosby Co., St. Louis, 1975, Chapter 25.

PAST MEDICAL HISTORY

One month prior to this hospitalization, Naomi Jackson, a 72-year-old woman, developed severe pain in her left lower jaw. She took two aspirins several times a day and this partially relieved the pain. She went to her dentist who diagnosed her problem as an abscessed molar and prescribed oral penicillin to reduce the infection, and propoxyphene (Darvon) to relieve the pain. The dentist stated that seven to fourteen days of antibiotic treatment would be necessary before he could extract the tooth. Within 48 hours, Mrs. Jackson began having tarry stools. Previous medical history revealed a healed duodenal ulcer. Mrs. Jackson had been hospitalized two times for the ulcer and had been treated medically. The dentist referred Mrs. Jackson for medical treatment.

Mrs. Jackson is a housewife and lives on a farm with her husband. Her husband was hospitalized three months prior to this time with congestive heart failure. Although Mr. Jackson's condition had improved, his wife has been concerned about him. They have two grown daughters who live near their parents. Mrs. Jackson is active in community and church affairs. She does not smoke or drink alcoholic beverages.

PRESENT HOSPITAL ADMISSION

Mrs. Jackson was seen at the clinic by her medical doctor. Her main complaints were weakness and having dark stools. During the physical examination, the doctor found that Mrs. Jackson had tenderness throughout the upper abdomen and epigastric area. Peristalsis was normal. The physician made the diagnosis of probable peptic ulcer and admitted Mrs. Jackson to the hospital.

First Hospital Day

4:00 P.M. When the nurse admitted Mrs. Jackson, she noted that the patient looked pale and weak.

Medical Orders

(1) Ulcer diet
(2) Milk 120 ml p.o. every 2 hours
(3) Magnesium hydroxide and aluminum hydroxide gel (Maalox) 8 ml p.o. every 2 hours (alternate with milk for administration every 1 hour)
(4) Propoxyphene (Darvon) 65 mg p.o. every 4 hours p.r.n. for pain
(5) Complete blood count in A.M.
(6) Hemoglobin and hematocrit every day
(7) Stool specimen for occult blood to laboratory every day
(8) Gastrointestinal series in A.M.
(9) Bedrest with bathroom privileges

Study Questions

1. Prior to hospitalization, Mrs. Jackson was taking aspirin, propoxyphene, and phenoxymethyl penicillin (Penicillin V). Could any of these drugs have reactivated the ulcer? If so, which one(s)?

2. What side effects of the drug(s) would have caused the ulcer to become active?

3. Explain how Mrs. Jackson could have minimized these adverse effects.

4. What relationships are possible between activation of the ulcer, the medications being taken, and other circumstances in Mrs. Jackson's life ?

5. Compare other treatments with medication administration in the management of Mrs. Jackson's peptic ulcer.

6. What is the purpose of milk in the medical regime?

7. Describe the action of magnesium hydroxide and aluminum hydroxide gel.

8. Magnesium hydroxide and aluminum hydroxide gel is a nonsystemic antacid. Compare the advantages and disadvantages of nonsystemic antacids with systemic antacids.

9. Antacids antagonize the action of some other drugs by decreasing the absorption of the other drugs in the alkaline pH caused by the antacids. What are some of these drugs?

10. What is the purpose of ordering the milk and the magnesium hydroxide and aluminum hydroxide gel to be given on alternate hours?

11. Describe the pharmacological action of propoxyphene and discuss its side effects.

12. How does the usual dose of propoxyphene compare with the dose ordered for Mrs. Jackson?

13. Explain why propoxyphene with aspirin would not be ordered as an analgesic

14. How can the results of the daily hemoglobin and hematocrit be used to evaluate the effectiveness or ineffectiveness of the medical treatment?

15. How can the results of the stool specimen be used to evaluate the effectiveness or ineffectiveness of the treatment?

5:00 P.M. Mrs. Jackson asked the nurse for medication for pain. She stated that both her left lower jaw and her stomach hurt. She had tears in her eyes and said she was worried because she had to be in the hospital and away from her husband, although she knew her daughters would help care for him. The nurse listened sympathetically to Mrs. Jackson and gave her propoxyphene 65 mg for her pain.

Study Questions

16. Explain what emotional factors may have caused Mrs. Jackson to need an analgesic at this particular time.

17. How could the supportive care given by the nurse enhance the effectiveness of the drug?

Second Hospital Day

9:00 A.M. The laboratory tests and x-ray studies were completed. When the nurse gave Mrs. Jackson the magnesium hydroxide and aluminum hydroxide gel, the patient asked for a glass of water. During the morning, the nurse began a care plan for Mrs. Jackson.

Laboratory and X-ray Results (4:00 P.M.)

Hemoglobin	10.3 gm/100 ml
Hematocrit	31%
Stool specimen for occult blood	4+

Gastrointestinal series showed a small ulcer on the posterior aspect of the duodenal bulb

Medical Orders

Propantheline bromide (Probanthine) 15 mg p.o. t.i.d. a.c.

Study Questions

18. What should the nurse teach the patient about drinking water with an antacid?

19. What relationship between medication administration and psychological support should the nurse consider in preparing a nursing care plan for Mrs. Jackson?

20. To what drug group does propantheline bromide belong?

21. What action of propantheline bromide makes it an appropriate medication for the treatment of a peptic ulcer?

22. What teaching should the nurse do in relationship to the side effects of propantheline bromide?

23. If Mrs. Jackson develops dryness of the mouth from taking propantheline bromide, what could the nurse suggest to help alleviate this side effect?

Fourth Hospital Day

9:00 A. M. Mrs Jackson had less abdominal pain during the last 24 hours, and she seemed more adjusted to her hospitalization. She still had some tenderness in the epigastric area and had occasional pain in the left lower jaw. Her stools were not as dark as they were previously. She told the nurse that an antacid she had taken during an earlier hospitalization had made her constipated.

Laboratory Results

Hemoglobin	10.4 gm/100 ml
Hematocrit	32%
Stool specimen for occult blood	1+

Medical Orders

Benzathine penicillin g (Bicillin) 600,000 units IM today

Study Questions

24. Compare the duration of action of benzathine penicillin g with that of other preparations of penicillin. Include the advantages of each.

25. Identify the side effects of penicillin that the nurse should watch for in Mrs. Jackson.

26. Describe the site and manner of administering an injection of benzathine penicillin g.

27. Considering the composition of magnesium hydroxide and aluminum hydroxide gel, explain what patient-instruction the nurse could do in relationship to Mrs. Jackson's remark about constipation.

Seventh Hospital Day

9:00 A.M. The nurse noted that Mrs. Jackson had not asked for an analgesic for three days. The patient said that the epigastric tenderness had subsided. She told the nurse that her husband sometimes took sodium bicarbonate to relieve indigestion.

Laboratory Results (4:00 P.M.)

Hemoglobin	10.7 gm/100 ml
Hematocrit	33%
Stool specimen for occult blood	trace

Medical Orders

(1) Up for 1 hour t.i.d.
(2) Discontinue milk and magnesium hydroxide and aluminum hydroxide gel (Maalox) from 10:00 P.M. to 6:00 A.M.

Study Questions

28. What nursing observation indicated effectiveness of the medical treatment for Mrs. Jackson's peptic ulcer?

29. How did the physician's orders indicate that the patient was improving with the treatment?

30. Discuss the action of sodium bicarbonate administration. What are the disadvantages of this medication? How should these disadvantages be discussed with Mrs. Jackson?

Tenth Hospital Day

11:00 A.M. Mrs. Jackson continued to be free of pain, and she was not as weak as she was at the time of admission. The stool specimen for occult blood had been negative for three days. The patient was discharged.

Discharge Orders

(1) Ulcer diet
(2) Milk, half glass between meals
(3) Magnesium hydroxide and aluminum hydroxide del (Maalox) 8 ml p.o. t.i.d. p.c.
(4) Ferrous gluconate (Fergon) 100 mg p.o. t.i.d. p.c.
(5) Return to the clinic for follow-up care in two weeks

Study Questions

31. Mrs. Jackson asked the nurse how long she would have to continue to take an antacid. What is an appropriate answer to her question?

32. Mrs. Jackson told the nurse she thought it would be more convenient for her to take antacid tablets rather than the liquid. Compare the advantages and disadvantages of the tablets with the liquid.

33. What are the pharmacological actions of ferrous gluconate? Why is it given after meals?

34. There may be a change in stool color while a person is taking an oral iron preparation. What change would the nurse tell Mrs. Jackson to expect?

35. Develop a teaching plan for Mrs. Jackson. Include the discharge medications as well as diet, rest, and activity.

REFERENCES

Antacids and ulcers. Hosp. Formulary Management, March, 1974, 23.

Crawford, F. A., et al.: Stress ulcer syndrome. R.N. 35:1-9, 1972.

Cupit, G. C., et al.: Antacids. Am. J. Nurs. 72:2210-2212, 1972.

Griffith, H. W.: Instructions for Patients. W. B. Saunders Co., Philadelphia, 1968, pp. 137-142.

Lambert, Jr., M. L.: Drug and diet interactions. Am. J. Nurs. 75:402-406, 1975.

Librach, I. M.: Peptic ulcer: facts and figures. Nurs. Mirror 134:23-24, 1972.

Lowenthal, W.: Programmed instruction: factors affecting drug absorption. Am. J. Nurs. 73:1391-1408, 1973.

Rodman, M. J.: Adjusting medications for the needs of the elderly. R.N. 38:65-89, 1975.

4

THE PATIENT WITH RHEUMATOID ARTHRITIS

TEXTBOOKS SUGGESTED FOR THIS STUDY

Asperheim, M. K., and Eisenhauer, L. A.: The Pharmacologic Basis of Patient Care, ed. 2. W. B. Saunders Co., Philadelphia, 1973, Chapters 11 and 17.

Bergersen, B.: Pharmacology in Nursing, ed. 13. C. V. Mosby Co., St. Louis, 1976, Chapters 11, 12, and 25.

Brunner, L. S., and Suddarth, D.: Textbook of Medical Surgical Nursing, ed. 3. J. B. Lippincott Co., Philadelphia, 1975, Chapter 36.

Goodman, L., and Gilman, A. (eds.): The Pharmacological Basis of Therapeutics, ed. 5. Macmillan Co., New York, 1975, Chapter 46.

Luckmann, J., and Sorensen, K.: Medical-Surgical Nursing — A Psychophysiologic Approach. W. B. Saunders Co., Philadelphia, 1974, Chapter 90.

Rodman, M. J., and Smith, D.: Pharmacology and Drug Therapy in Nursing. J. B. Lippincott Co., Philadelphia, 1974, Chapters 10, 16, and 22.

Shafer, K. N., et al.: Medical Surgical Nursing, ed. 6. C. V. Mosby Co., St.Louis, 1975, Chapter 33.

PAST MEDICAL HISTORY

Mrs. Jones, a 73-year-old widow, had an eleven-year history of rheumatoid arthritis. At the time that the diagnosis was made, she was hospitalized and given a brief course of steroid therapy. When she was discharged she was advised to take aspirin for pain and swelling. She and her husband had lived in a mobile home and he had cared for her until his death. When he died it was necessary for Mrs. Jones to move to a home for disabled persons. She had two married daughters who had families of their own. They visited her in the home and helped with her care. Her condition had become worse during recent years.

PRESENT HOSPITAL ADMISSION

First Hospital Day

Mrs. Jones was admitted to the hospital at 5:00 P.M. For several days prior she had severe pain in her right hip, and the attendant at the home was unable to get her out of bed. During admission, she stated that the arthritis had started in her left hand and gradually affected both hands and feet. The nurse observed that movement was severly restricted in the patient's wrists, elbows, ankles, and knees. The physician made the diagnosis of chronic, generalized, and advanced rheumatoid arthritis.

Medical Orders

(1) Regular diet
(2) Indomethacin (Indocin) 25 mg p.o. t.i.d.
(3) Diazepam (Valium) 2 mg p.o. t.i.d.
(4) Aspirin, aluminum dihydroxyaminoacetate and magnesium carbonate (Bufferin) 600 mg every 4 hours p.r.n.
(5) Complete blood count, erythrosedimentation rate, hemoglobin, hematocrit, rheumatoid arthritis factor, lupus erythematosus prep, and reticulocyte count
(6) Urinalysis
(7) X-ray hands, wrists, elbows, shoulders, hips, knees, ankles; and lumbar, sacral, and cervical spine

Study Questions

1. What specific action of indomethacin makes it effective in the treatment of rheumatoid arthritis?

2. Considering the adverse effects caused by indomethacin, explain the time schedule the nurse would use to administer it.

3. Indomethacin has the potential of causing serious adverse effects. What signs and symptoms of such effects would the nurse look for as she cares for Mrs. Jones?

4. How is the psychotropic action of diazepam useful to the emotional adjustment of persons with chronic illness?

5. What other therapeutic action of diazepam makes it a drug of choice in the treatment of rheumatoid arthritis?

6. Which of the possible etiological factors in rheumatoid arthritis are related to the administration of a tranquilizer such as diazepam?

7. Adrenocorticoid steroids were previously used in the treatment of arthritis. Their discontinuance was related to their toxic effects and severe rebound phenomena following withdrawal. Discuss both of these effects.

8. How does the difference in the composition of aspirin with dihydroxyaminoacetate and magnesium carbonate and plain aspirin account for the difference in their side effects?

9. Why are narcotic analgesics not used routinely to treat a patient with a chronic illness?

10. What is the danger in treating chronic pain with aspirin without consulting a physician?

Second Hospital Day

8:30 A.M. The nurse who bathed Mrs. Jones noted that her fingers were swollen. Mrs. Jones complained of pain and the nurse gave her the analgesic.

Laboratory Results (9:30 A.M.)

White blood count	5000 per cu mm
Hemoglobin	11.2 gm/100 ml
Hematocrit	34%
Erythrosedimentation rate	55 mm/hr
Reticulocyte count	1%
Rheumatoid arthritis factor	positive
Lupus erythematosus prep	no lupus erythematosus cells seen
Urinalysis	clear, straw-colored
pH	acid
specific gravity	1.021
albumin	negative
sugar	negative
acetone	negative
white blood cell	occasional
epithelium	occasional
X-ray results	confirmed ankylosing rheumatoid arthritis

1:00 P.M. Mrs. Jones appeared comfortable and did not complain of pain following administration of the analgesic at 9:00 A.M. At 1:00 P.M. she complained of pain in the right hip and the nurse repeated the analgesic. Mrs. Jones told the nurse that when she was first hospitalized for arthritis she was given some pills that helped her very much, and she asked why she couldn't take them all the time. From the description of the medicine, the nurse understood that she was talking about a medication of the steroid group.

9:00 P.M. When the nurse prepared Mrs. Jones for bed, she positioned her in order to give support to the inflamed joints. She also arranged the bed covers to avoid any localized pressure. Mrs. Jones said she could not go to sleep because of the pain in her hip. The nurse gave her the analgesic.

Study Questions

11. What explanation would the nurse give Mrs. Jones regarding the use of steroid therapy?

12. What other measures besides the analgesic did the nurse use to relieve pain?

Fourth Hospital Day

9:00 A.M. Mrs. Jones complained of less pain. The nurse noted that the patient had increased range of motion at the elbows as she gave her a bath and changed her gown.

Medical Orders

(1) Hot packs to painful joints b.i.d.
(2) Exercises by physiotherapy b.i.d.
(3) Magnesium hydroxide with aluminum hydroxide gel (Maalox) 4 ml t.i.d. to be administered with indomethacin (Indocin)

The physical therapist instigated a program of active range of motion exercises for the upper extremities and active assistive exercises for the lower extremities.

Study Questions

13. What indications are there that the medications Mrs. Jones has received are effective?

14. What is the relationship of the other modes of therapy ordered to the drugs being used?

15. What explanation should the nurse give the patient for taking magnesium hydroxide with aluminum hydroxide gel along with the indomethacin?

Ninth Hospital Day

9:00 A.M. Mrs. Jones' joints continued to be swollen and stiff, but she was able to do more of her own care. She did not complain of nausea or indigestion and the analgesic controlled her pain. She usually needed the analgesic twice a day. The nurse suggested she take it prior to receiving physiotherapy, and the patient requested it at bedtime.

Medical Orders

(1) White blood count, hemoglobin, and hematocrit
(2) Urinalysis

Study Questions

16. What evidence indicates continued effectiveness of indomethacin?

17. Is indomethacin being tolerated satisfactorily? Why?

18. How did the nurse use the drug therapy to increase the effectiveness of the physiotherapy?

Tenth Hospital Day

Laboratory Results (9:30 A.M.)

White blood count	6500 per cu mm
Hemoglobin	12 gm/100 ml
Hematocrit	36%

Urinalysis	clear, straw-colored
pH	acid
specific gravity	1.022
albumin	negative
sugar	negative
acetone	negative
white blood cells	occasional

Medical Orders

Gold sodium thiomalate (Myochrysine) 10 mg IM today

The nurse administered the gold sodium thiomalate and requested that the patient lie in a recumbent position following the injection.

Study Questions

19. Describe the therapeutic action of gold sodium thiomalate as related to the pathophysiology of rheumatoid arthritis.

20. Why did the physician order a white blood count, hemoglobin, hematocrit, and urinalysis prior to ordering the gold sodium thiomalate?

21. The possibility of a toxic reaction from the adverse effects of gold injections should always be explained to the patient before the injections are begun. What are the most common signs and symptoms of these effects?

22. Describe the usual schedule for administration of gold sodium thiomalate.

23. Mrs. Jones asked the nurse when to expect an improvement in her condition as a result of the gold shots. Considering the schedule of administering these injections, what would be the appropriate reply?

24. In addition to laboratory results, what nursing assessments are of value in identifying toxic reactions to gold sodium thiomalate?

25. Why did the nurse ask the patient to lie in a recumbent position following administration of the gold?

Summary of First Month's Hospitalization

In the month following admission, Mrs. Jones made slow but gradual improvement. She was able to take a more active part in the exercises done by physiotherapy. She could also get from the wheel chair to the commode with help rather than having to use the bedpan. The swelling in her fingers decreased. She received gold sodium thiomalate 15 mg the third week, and 25 mg the fourth week after admission. She was then transferred to the extended care facility connected with the hospital. She was sad to leave the surroundings to which she had become accustomed. The nurse went with her when she was transferred and promised to visit her there. The physician planned to continue the same medical regime.

First Week in the Extended Care Facility

During the first week in the extended care facility, Mrs. Jones experienced nausea and on two occasions she vomited a small amount of undigested food.

Study Questions

27. Which of the medications would the nurse suspect to be causing the nausea?

28. What is the nurse's responsibility when she believes that a medication is causing nausea and vomiting?

29. What other circumstances could be causing Mrs. Jones to have nausea and vomiting?

Second Week in the Extended Care Facility

The nurses in the extended care facility worked out a nursing care plan to help Mrs. Jones in her adjustment to her new environment. As she became more accustomed to the new environment, the nausea and vomiting subsided and she was able to continue with the medical regime.

Summary of Second Month of Care

At the end of two months, the nurse noted that Mrs. Jones was better able to move her extremities. She could not move her hips enough to walk, but she could stand with help. She did not have any increase in the motion of her knees. The nursing staff assisted with exercises between physiotherapy visits. Mrs. Jones said she could move all of her extremities more than when she was admitted, and she was especially pleased to be able to straighten her fingers. She did not complain of indigestion, nor did she have any skin rashes. The gold sodium thiomalate was increased to 50 mg every week. The physician ordered a check of the patient's white blood cells, hemoglobin, hematocrit, platelets, erythrosedimentation rate, and urine every week prior to the administration of the gold injections.

<u>Laboratory Results</u>

White blood count	4000 per cu mm
Hemoglobin	9 gm/100 ml
Hematocrit	28%
Platelets	80,000
Erythrosedimentation rate	36 mm/hr
Urinalysis	cloudy, straw-colored
pH	acid
specific gravity	1.025
albumin	1+
sugar	negative
acetone	negative
white blood cells	3-6
bacteria	few
epithelium	few

Medical Orders

Omit gold sodium thiomalate (Myochrysine) this week

Study Questions

30. What are the possible reasons why gold sodium thiomalate was omitted?

31. What signs and symptoms does the nurse need to observe related to the above laboratory results?

32. What would be an appropriate explanation for the nurse to give Mrs. Jones as to why she did not receive the gold injection?

Summary of Third Month of Care

At the end of three months Mrs. Jones could not walk but was able to roll herself in the wheelchair. This added to her feeling of independence. Her blood count and urinalysis returned to normal. She remained in the extended care facility. The physician planned to continue the same medical regime with a maintenance dose of gold sodium thiomalate 50 mg once a month.

Study Questions

33. What evidence should the nurse continue to evaluate to determine the effectiveness or ineffectiveness of Mrs. Jones' treatment?

REFERENCES

Drakontides, A.: Drugs to treat pain. Am. J. Nurs., 74:508-513, 1974.

Driscoll, P. W.: Rheumatoid arthritis: managing it more successfully. Nursing '75, 5:29-32, 1975.

Driscoll, P. W.: Rheumatoid arthritis: understanding it more fully. Nursing '75, 5:26-28, 1975.

Duff, I. F., et al.: Comprehensive management of patients with rheumatoid arthritis. Arthritis Rheum., 17:635-645, 1974.

Goth, A.: Medical Pharmacology, ed. 6. C. V. Mosby Co., St. Louis, 1973.

Loxley, A. K.: The emotional toll of crippling deformity. Am. J. Nurs., 72:1839-1840, 1972.

Macrae, I.: Arthritis: its nature and management. Nurs. Clin. N. Am., 8:643-652, 1973.

Mowat, A. G., and Davies, L.: Rheumatoid arthritis: some aspects of current medical treatment. Part I. Nurs. Times, 71:1400-1401, 1975.

Murray, R., and Zentner, J.: Guidelines for more effective health teaching. Nursing '76, 6:44-53, 1976.

Pitorak, E.: Rheumatoid arthritis: living with it more comfortably. Nursing '75, 5:33-35, 1975.

Rodman, M. J.: Drugs for treating anxiety. R.N., 36:57-58, 1973.

Cooperating Clinics Committee of Am. Rheumatoid Assn. A controlled trial of gold salt therapy in rheumatoid arthritis. Arthritis Rheum., 16:353-358, 1973.

5

THE PATIENT WITH CHRONIC RENAL FAILURE

TEXTBOOKS SUGGESTED FOR THIS STUDY

Asperheim, M. K., and Eisenhauer, L. A.: Pharmacologic Basis of Patient Care, ed. 2. W. B. Saunders Co., Philadelphia, 1973, Chapters 6, 9, 13, and 19.

Bergersen, B.: Pharmacology in Nursing, ed. 13. C. V. Mosby Co., St. Louis, 1976, Chapters 10, 19, and 20.

Brunner, L. S., and Suddarth, D.: Textbook of Medical Surgical Nursing, ed. 3. J. B. Lippincott Co., Philadelphia, 1975, Chapter 26.

Goodman, L., and Gilman, A. (eds.): The Pharmacological Basis of Therapeutics, ed. 5. Macmillan Co., New York, 1975, Chapters 33, 39, 56, and 61.

Luckmann, J., and Sorensen, K.: Medical-Surgical Nursing — A Psychophysiologic Approach. W. B. Saunders Co., Philadelphia, 1974, Chapters 55, 56, 57, and 58.

Rodman, M. J., and Smith, D.: Pharmacology and Drug Therapy in Nursing. J. B. Lippincott Co., Philadelphia, 1974, Chapter 41.

Shafer, K. N., et al.: Medical Surgical Nursing, ed. 6. C. V. Mosby Co., St. Louis, 1975, Chapter 20.

PAST MEDICAL HISTORY

Mr. Cortez, a 39-year-old man, has had a three-year history of chronic glomerulonephritis with hypertension. Initially, Mr. Cortez sought medical help because of a persistent upper respiratory infection. At that time the physician learned that Mr. Cortez had had a cold four weeks prior to seeking medical assistance, had felt very tired, and had continuous headaches. Preliminary studies were scheduled and revealed the following: albuminuria, hypertension (blood pressure 170/100), slight azotemia, and a urine culture that was positive for Escherichia coli. His excretory urogram (IVP) was normal.

A diagnosis of acute glomerulonephritis was made. Mr. Cortez was treated on an outpatient basis.

<u>Medical Orders</u>

(1) Sulfisoxazole (Gantrisin) 500 mg 4 tablets initially followed by 2 tablets q.i.d. for 2 weeks
(2) Hydrochlorothiazide (Oretic) 100 mg daily
(3) Hydralazine hydrochloride (Apresoline) 10 mg q.i.d. p.c. and h.s.

(4) Liberal fluid intake

Study Questions

1. What is the action of sulfisoxazole? Discuss the reason for its administration to Mr. Cortez. Since Mr. Cortez is being given sulfisoxazole on an outpatient basis, how can he evaluate the effectiveness of this medication? What patient teaching needs to be done by the nurse in relation to this?

2. What is the rationale for encouraging a liberal fluid intake when Mr. Cortez was placed on sulfisoxazole? In relation to a 24-hour time period, define what a liberal fluid intake would be.

3. The Stevens-Johnson syndrome can occur with patients receiving sulfisoxazole. What is this syndrome? What signs and/or symptoms does Mr. Cortez need to be alert to in relation to this syndrome? What should Mr. Cortez do if he shows any of these signs and/or symptoms?

4. What other side and toxic effects might Mr. Cortez encounter with sulfisoxazole?

5. Hydrochlorothiazide has been ordered for Mr. Cortez. Describe its action as an antihypertensive agent.

6. What are the other actions of hydrochlorothiazide?

7. Hydrochlorothiazide sometimes causes a diabetes mellitus effect. Explain why this occurs. What signs and/or symptoms would indicate that this has occurred with Mr. Cortez?

8. If diabetes mellitus symptoms occur in Mr. Cortez, how can the effects of these symptoms be reversed, or will Mr. Cortez be diabetic permanently?

9. Hyponatremia is one of the electrolyte imbalances that may occur in Mr. Cortez. Since hydrochlorothiazide was administered on an outpatient basis, what signs and/or symptoms should the nurse tell Mr. Cortez he should be alert to in relation to hyponatremia? If these signs or symptoms occur, what should Mr. Cortez do?

10. Hypokalemia is another electrolyte imbalance that Mr. Cortez may encounter. What indications of this condition would be important for Mr. Cortez to be alert to? Is there anything that Mr. Cortez could do on an outpatient basis that would minimize this condition from occuring?

PRESENT HOSPITAL ADMISSION

First Hospital Day

Mr. Cortez' initial response to treatment on an outpatient basis was excellent and he remained in good health for three years. Then he developed nausea, vomiting, anorexia, and diarrhea which persisted for one week. An appointment with his physician resulted in an immediate hospital admission.

Vital signs on admission were temperature 101° F., pulse 100, respirations 32, and blood pressure 180/110. Weight on admission was 177 pounds.

Laboratory Results

White blood cell count	8300 per cu mm
Hematocrit	38.5%
Hemoglobin	12.9 gm/100 ml
Urinalysis	Straw-colored
Specific gravity	1.012
pH	5.0
Albumin	3+
White blood cells	many
Hyaline	1-4
Casts	1-2
Sugar	2+
Acetone	negative
Bacteria	4+

Admitting Diagnoses

(1) Hypertensive cardiovascular disease
(2) Renal failure
(3) Rule out early congestive heart failure
(4) Urinary tract infection

Medical Orders

(1) Urine for culture and sensitivity now
(2) 40 gm protein diet
(3) Up ad lib.
(4) Intake and output
(5) Blood pressure and pulse every hour until stable, then every 4 hours
(6) Weigh daily
(7) Laboratory work
   Blood urea nitrogen
   Creatinine
   Uric acid
   24-hour urine for creatinine
   Electrolytes: sodium, potassium, chloride, bicarbonate
   Fasting blood glucose
(8) Medications
   Colistimethate sodium (Coly-Mycin M) 200 mg IM b.i.d. to begin after urine for culture and sensitivity obtained
   Methyldopa (Aldomet) 250 mg p.o. q.i.d.
   Hydralazine hydrochloride (Apresoline) 10 mg p.o. q.i.d.
   Reserpine (Serpasil) 0.1 mg p.o. b.i.d.
   Reserpine (Serpasil) 1.25 mg IM stat.
   Trimethobenzamide (Tigan) 100 mg IM every 4 hours p.r.n. nausea, give 1 dose now

Acetaminophen (Tylenol) 600 mg every 4 hours p.r.n. for oral temperature elevated above 101° F.

(9) IV therapy: 1000 ml 5% dextrose in 0.2% saline with 2 ml vitamin B and C (Berocca C) to run at 75 ml/hour. Repeat IV order when first IV is completed.

(10) Electrocardiogram now

Study Questions

11. Prior to giving Mr. Cortez the colistimethate, the nurse should ask whether he has any allergies. If Mr. Cortez indicates he has any allergies, what should the nurse do?

12. Why has colistimethate been ordered for Mr. Cortez? Against what type of organisms is it effective? What are its actions?

13. What effect does colistimethate have on the renal system? How will its excretion be affected by Mr. Cortez' diagnosis?

14. How is the dose of colistimethate calculated? Is Mr. Cortez receiving an average dose? Give the rationale for your answer.

15. What important nursing measures will need to be implemented as a result of Mr. Cortez' being on colistimethate? What toxic effects may Mr. Cortez encounter as a result of being on colistimethate?

16. What effect might the medications ordered for Mr. Cortez have on the electrocardiogram?

17. What is the action of reserpine and why has it been ordered to be given stat. for Mr. Cortez? Define stat. and discuss how medications ordered this way are administered

18. What is the average dose of reserpine? Compare the amount of medication ordered for the stat. dose versus that ordered for the daily dose. Explain the rationale for the difference in dosage.

19. Compare the actions of methyldopa, hydralazine, and reserpine and discuss how each is effective in the treatment of Mr. Cortez' condition. Why were all of these medications ordered for Mr. Cortez?

20. What side and toxic effects does the nurse need to be alert to in relation to the antihypertensive medications Mr. Cortez is receiving? How long will it be before the side and/or toxic effects may manifest themselves?

21. Methyldopa is absorbed by the gastrointestinal tract and excreted by the kidneys. How will this affect Mr. Cortez' serum electrolytes and acid/base balance? How will the absorption of methyldopa be affected as a result of the vomiting and diarrhea that Mr. Cortez is experiencing?

22. What criteria should the nurse use in evaluating the effects of the administration of methyldopa, hydralazine, and reserpine on Mr. Cortez?

Second Hospital Day

Mr. Cortez was restless during the afternoon and evening of the first day. Although his respirations were increased they were not labored, and Mr. Cortez experienced dyspnea only on exertion. He was medicated with trimethobenzemide twice during the first 24 hours, once upon admission and once during the night. He experienced no vomiting. His temperature remained elevated between 100° and 101° F. The urine for culture and sensitivity was obtained after which the 24-hour urine was started. Mr. Cortez, who was weighed before breakfast, was 176 pounds. His blood pressure ranged between 170-176/100-110. His pulse averaged 88 (radial) and 92 (apical). His restlessness decreased.

Study Questions

23. What indications are there of the effectiveness of trimethobenzemide during the first 24 hours of Mr. Cortez' hospitalization?

24. Reye's syndrome is associated with the use of trimethobenzemide. What is this syndrome? Has Mr. Cortez experienced any of the signs and/or symptoms associated with this syndrome?

Third Hospital Day

Mr. Cortez' nausea and vomiting subsided but the problems with anorexia continued. Diarrhea continued but decreased in amount. His blood pressure averaged 158/100 lying down and 140/88 standing. His weight was 175 pounds.

Laboratory Results

Blood urea nitrogen	93 mg/100 ml
Creatinine	13.2 mg/100 ml
Electrolytes	
Sodium	139 mEq/L
Potassium	4.2 mEq/L
Chloride	102 mEq/L
Bicarbonate	21 mEq/L
Uric acid	10.0 mg/100 ml
24-hour urine for creatinine	
Total volume	2940
Creatinine	1.0 gm/24 hours (Normal 0.7-2.0 gm/24 hours)

Mr. Cortez complained of being tired all the time and had several bouts of dizziness when ambulating. As a result of the dizziness, Mr. Cortez was placed on bedrest with bathroom privileges. A 48-hour report on the urine culture and sensitivity indicated that Mr. Cortez had a Pseudomonus aeruginosa infection which was sensitive to colistimethate. Total intake for Mr. Cortez was 2000 ml and output was 2940 ml.

Study Questions

25. What is the relationship between dizziness and the medications that Mr. Cortez is taking? What nursing measures should be employed in relation to Mr. Cortez' dizziness?

26. What are the possible reasons why diuretics have not been ordered for Mr. Cortez?

27. Sodium polystyrene sulfonate is a commonly used cation-exchange resin. Where does the action of polystyrene sulfonate take place? Why is this site of action especially important in the treatment of patients with renal failure? Based on Mr. Cortez' initial electrolyte laboratory results, what changes might you expect if Mr. Cortez were placed on polystyrene sulfonate?

28. Eighth cranial nerve damage can occur with one of the medications Mr. Cortez is taking. Which medication is this? What signs and/or symptoms will Mr. Cortez display if eighth cranial nerve damage has occurred?

29. If eighth cranial nerve damage were to occur in Mr. Cortez, would the effects of the damage be reversible when the medication was discontinued?

Fourth Hospital Day

Mr. Cortez became increasingly irritable, had difficulty carrying on a conversation, and was having difficulty sleeping at night. The nurse noted that Mr. Cortez' skin had a yellowish tinge and he frequently scratched his skin. Although Mr. Cortez had not gained any weight, his blood pressure was increasing, sometimes running as high as 186/120. His pulse remained between 80 and 88. Total urine output decreased to 600 ml in the previous 24 hours. The physician ordered a Foley catheter to be inserted and hourly urines to be done.

Laboratory Results

Blood urea nitrogen	110 mg/100 ml
Creatinine	15.7 mg/100 ml
Uric acid	8.4 mg/100 ml

Study Questions

30. Reserpine is a sympathetic blocking agent. Are any of the symptoms Mr. Cortez is experiencing related to the effects that result from sympathetic fibers being blocked?

31. If vomiting should reoccur in the future, to which medications might it be related?

32. What information will help to evaluate whether Mr. Cortez' skin irritation is due to a sensitivity to medications or to pathological changes?

Fifth to Eighth Hospital Days

While he was on conservative medical management, there was no significant improvement in Mr. Cortez' uremic state. His blood urea nitrogen continued to increase as did his uric acid level. Output ranged between 100 and 600 ml in 24 hours. Although his urinary tract infection had been controlled and his temperature was within normal range, his blood pressure remained elevated, running between 170-186/110-120. Mr. Cortez' physician spoke with Mr. Cortez and his wife and explained his plan to prepare Mr. Cortez for hemodialysis. The creation of an arteriovenous shunt was scheduled for the next day.

Ninth Hospital Day

Mr. Cortez had his first hemodialysis treatment and his weight dropped eight pounds. His blood pressure lying down ranged between 100-120/66-70. He continued to complain of tiredness and headaches. The skin itching decreased and the yellow skin coloring disappeared.

Within a week the physician discharged Mr. Cortez. He was to continue with hemodialysis treatments three times a week.

Discharge Orders

(1) Guanethidine sulfate (Ismelin) 50 mg p.o. daily
(2) Hydralazine hydrochloride (Apresoline) 25 mg p.o. t.i.d.
(3) Vitamin B complex with C (Folbesyn) 1 tablet b.i.d.
(4) Ferrous sulfate 300 mg p.o. t.i.d.

Study Questions

33. Could Mr. Cortez' headaches have been related to any of the medications he was receiving? If so, which ones?

34. What is the action of guanethidine? What is the site of its action? What are the side and toxic effects of guanethidine about which the nurse should inform Mr. Cortez?

35. Develop a teaching plan in relation to the discharge medications Mr. Cortez is receiving.

36. How should Mr. Cortez be taught to evaluate the effectiveness of these medications at home?

37. What side effects should Mr. Cortez be alert to in relation to these medications?

38. When on hemodialysis, patients are usually placed on vitamins. Why does Mr. Cortez require vitamin supplementation? What kind of vitamin supplementation is needed? Why?

39. What is the relationship between the anemia associated with renal failure and the administration of iron therapy?

40. What does Mr. Cortez need to be taught regarding his anemia and iron therapy? How does iron affect the gastrointestinal system? What measures can be taken to decrease these side effects?

41. Mr. Cortez' antihypertensive medications were decreased when he was discharged. What advantages and disadvantages are there in the treatment of hypertension with fluids and sodium restriction when a patient is on hemodialysis rather than with a large dosage of hypertensive medications?

42. What is the effect of antihypertensive medications on the libido?

REFERENCES

Corea, A. L.: Current trends in diet and drug therapy for the dialysis patient. Nurs. Clin. N. Am. 10:469-479, 1975.

Davis, J. E.: Drugs for urologic disorders. Am. J. Nurs. 65:107-112, 1965.

Dipalma, J. R.: Preventing drug toxicity in renal failure. R.N. 38:65-69, 1975.

Dolan, P. O., and Greene, H. L.: Renal failure and peritoneal dialysis. Nursing '75, 5:40-49, 1975.

Downing, S. R.: Nursing support in early renal failure. Am. J. Nurs. 69:1212-1216, 1969.

Long, M., Winslow, E., Scheubing, M., and Callahan, J.: Hypertension — what patients need to know. Am. J. Nurs. 76:765-770, 1976.

Schneider, W. J., and Boyce, B. A.: Complications of diuretic therapy. Am. J. Nurs. 68:1903-1907, 1968.

6

THE PATIENT WITH A KIDNEY TRANSPLANT

TEXTBOOKS SUGGESTED FOR THIS STUDY

Asperheim, M. K., and Eisenhauer, L. A.: The Pharmacologic Basis of Patient Care, ed. 2. W. B. Saunders Co., Philadelphia, 1973, Chapters 6, 7, 15, 17, 19, and 20.
Bergersen, B. S.: Pharmacology in Nursing, ed. 13. C. V. Mosby Co., St. Louis, 1976, Chapters 17, 19, 24, 25, and 31.
Brunner, L. S., and Suddarth, D.: Textbook of Medical Surgical Nursing, ed. 3. J. B. Lippincott Co., Philadelphia, 1975, Chapter 26.
Goodman, L., and Gilman, A. (eds.): The Pharmacological Basis of Therapeutics, ed. 5. Macmillan Co., New York, 1975, Chapters 29, 33, 36, 39, 48, 57, and 62.
Luckmann, J., and Sorensen, K.: Medical-Surgical Nursing — A Psychophysiologic Approach. W. B. Saunders Co., Philadelphia, 1974, Chapters 55, 56, 57, and 58.
Rodman, M. J., and Smith, D.: Pharmacology and Drug Therapy in Nursing. J. B. Lippincott Co., Philadelphia, 1974, Chapters 13, 14, 17, 18, 27, 45, and 48.
Shafer, K. N., et al.: Medical Surgical Nursing, ed. 6. C. V. Mosby Co., St. Louis, 1975, Chapter 20.

PAST MEDICAL HISTORY

Gary Wong, a 20-year-old university student, experienced no major medical difficulties until he broke his right arm while playing basketball one afternoon at the university gym. Gary was taken to the physician's office where a cast was applied. At that time, the physician did routine laboratory work. The results of the urinalysis indicated an abundant number of red blood cells. The history revealed that Gary had noticed some swelling of his eyes for the last four to five months, and he had also noted some hematuria. The physician admitted Gary to the hospital for further tests and treatment.

A kidney biopsy indicated that Gary had chronic sclerosing glomerulonephritis and he was placed on spironolactone with hydrochlorothiazide (Aldactazide), ampicillin, and sodium bicarbonate, and treated on an outpatient basis. One month later, Gary was readmitted to the hospital because of 1+ pedal edema and a fifteen-pound weight loss. Physical findings were within normal range except for Gary's blood pressure which was 130/96 mm Hg and a pulse rate of 124.

During Gary's second hospital stay, he had mild headaches and his blood pressure ranged between 110-150 mm Hg systolic, and 60-110 mm Hg diastolic. During this hospitalization, Gary was started on hydralazine hydrochloride (Apresoline) 25 mg p.o. t.i.d. because of hypertension. Because of poor renal function, an arteriovenous fistula was done on the left arm and he was started on hemodialysis.

Eventually Gary was discharged with diet instructions for a 40-gm protein no-added-salt diet, hydralazine 25 mg p.o. t.i.d., and instructions to clean and dress the arteriovenous fistula site daily. He was maintained on hemodialysis for three years. During that time, he developed problems with his first fistula and a second fistula was created in the right arm. While Gary was on the hemodialysis program, discussions of a kidney transplant took place with Gary and his family. Gary's mother offered to donate a kidney, and tissue typing was done. A suitable match was revealed, and plans for the kidney transplant were made.

PRESENT HOSPITAL ADMISSION

First Hospital Day

Gary was admitted to the hospital at 2:30 P.M. and scheduled for a heterotropic renal allotransplantation. The prospective donor was Gary's mother, Mrs. Wong. The typing match was AB which was an acceptable match since Gary had type B+ and Mrs. Wong O+.

At the time of admission, Gary's vital signs were temperature 99° F., pulse 96, respirations 18, and blood pressure 160/100. His weight was 105 pounds and he was 64 inches tall.

Medical Orders

(1) Diet: 1 gm sodium-modified low-potassium diet
(2) Hemodialysis tomorrow
(3) Weigh patient daily in A.M. before breakfast
(4) Blood pressure every 8 hours
(5) Laboratory studies
    Red blood cell count
    Hemoglobin
    Hematocrit
    Platelet count
    White blood cell count with differential
    Bilirubin
    Blood urea nitrogen
    Creatinine
    Glucose
    Total protein
    Albumin
    Uric acid
    SGOT
    Electrolytes: serum chloride, bicarbonate, potassium, and sodium
    Absolute lymphocyte count
(6) Medications:
    Magaldrate (Riopan) 15 ml every 2 hours while awake
    Acetaminophen (Tylenol) 2 tablets every 4 hours p.r.n. for rectal temperature above 103° F.
    Hydralazine hydrochloride (Apresoline) 25 mg b.i.d.

(7) Have available on the floor:
Epinephrine (Adrenalin) 1:1000
Diphenhydramine hydrochloride (Benadryl) for intravenous use
Methylprednisolone sodium succinate (Solu-Medrol) for intravenous use
(8) Crossmatch for one unit electrolyte poor red blood cells; have for tomorrow A.M.

Study Questions

1. What is the action of magaldrate and why has it been ordered for Gary?

2. What is the relationship between the action of magaldrate and the acid-base status of the body?

3. Gary has been on hydralazine for about three years. How is the action of this medication related to Gary's renal function? Can Gary's renal function be expected to improve as a result of the administration of hydralazine?

4. What is the relationship between the administration of magaldrate and hydralazine?

5. What is the action of epinephrine and methylprednisolone? Why have they been ordered to be available? Describe how these medications are prepared and administered.

Second Hospital Day

Laboratory Results

Red blood cell count		2.3 million per cu mm
Hemoglobin		7.3 gm/100 ml
Hematocrit		21.5%
White blood cell count		8,500 per cu mm
(differential)		
Segs	69%	
Lymphocytes	14%	
Monocytes	9%	
Eosinophils	7%	
Basophils	1%	
Bilirubin		0.4 mg/100 ml
Blood urea nitrogen		40 mg/100 ml
Creatinine		8.6 mg/100 ml
Glucose		109 mg/100 ml
Total protein		6.8 gm/100 ml
Albumin		3.6 gm/100 ml
Uric acid		7.7 mg/100 ml
SGOT		8 units
Chloride		98 mEq/L
Bicarbonate		24 mEq/L
Potassium		4.5 mEq/L
Sodium		138 mEq/L
Absolute lymphocyte count		1,150/cu mm

Gary spent most of the day receiving his hemodialysis treatment. The remainder of the day was uneventful with the exception of Gary's complaints of continued tiredness. Nursing care was planned around providing long periods of rest for him.

Third Hospital Day

Gary was scheduled for surgery in three days. Preoperative preparation was begun.

Medical Orders

(1) Diphenhydramine hydrochloride (Benadryl) 25 mg p.o. t.i.d.
(2) Azathioprine (Imuran) 150 mg p.o. in A.M.

Gary felt better. His weight had dropped by 3 pounds following the dialysis treatment, and his vital signs remained stable with no temperature elevation. Gary received a unit of electrolyte-poor red blood cells after which his laboratory studies were as follows:

Red blood cell count	3.0 million per cu mm
Hemoglobin	9.4 gm/100 ml
Hematocrit	27.5%
Platelet count	226,000 per cu mm
Blood urea nitrogen	55 mg/100 ml
Creatinine	9.3 mg/100 ml
Absolute lymphocyte count	1,478 per cu mm

White blood cell count was slightly elevated

Study Questions

6. What is the drug classification of azathioprine? What is the action of azathioprine in the body?

7. Why was azathioprine administered orally? Through what system is it excreted from the body? Considering Gary's diagnosis, how will its excretion be affected?

8. What nursing observations should the nurse consider since Gary is on azathioprine? What side effects might Gary experience?

9. It is important to continue frequent complete blood counts, platelet counts, and uric acid levels while Gary is on azathioprine. Why?

10. Liver function studies will also be important. Why? Which liver function studies would you expect to be ordered for Gary?

11. If a patient on azathioprine is also on allopurinol, the dose of azathioprine would have to be altered. Discuss how and why the dose would be altered.

12. What is the drug classification of diphenhydramine? What is its action? Why was it ordered for Gary preoperatively?

13. What are the side effects of diphenhydramine? What nursing observations can differentiate the side effects of diphenhydramine from the signs and symptoms of renal failure?

14. What is the rationale for the administration of diphenhydramine and azathioprine together?

Fourth Hospital Day

Gary received the diphenhydramine and azathioprine. He also received another unit of electrolyte-poor whole blood. His weight was 102 pounds. Daily blood work indicated a decrease in blood urea nitrogen and creatinine following each hemodialysis treatment. Gary had fewer complaints of being tired and his red blood cell count, hematocrit, and hemoglobin showed a slight increase. He was anxious about the surgery which was scheduled for the next day. Mrs. Wong was admitted to the hospital during the afternoon and was located in the room adjacent to Gary's.

Medical Orders

(1) Soap suds enema tonight
(2) Abdomino-pubic prep
(3) PhisoHex bath after soap suds enema and abdomino-pubic prep
(4) Daily blood work in A.M.
(5) NPO after midnight except for medication up until 3 hours preoperatively
    (surgery approximately 8:30 A.M.)
(6) Type and cross match for 4 units of fresh whole blood for OR in A.M.
(7) Preoperative medications: IM at 7:15 A.M.
    Meperidine hydrochloride (Demerol) 50 mg
    Atropine sulfate 0.4 mg
    Hydroxyzine hydrochloride (Vistaril) 50 mg
(8) Azathioprine (Imuran) 100 mg at 11:00 P.M. tonight

Study Questions

15. What nursing care should be given to Gary prior to administration of the preoperative medications? Why?

16. The preoperative medications have been ordered to be given to Gary at 7:15 A.M. When will the medications take effect? Compare the intramuscular, subcutaneous, and intravenous routes for administration of medications and identify why the intramuscular route was ordered for Gary's preoperative injection.

17. What is the action of each of the preoperative medications? Describe the rationale for giving all of the medications at the same time. Which of the medications can be mixed? Describe the procedure which should be used when mixing the preoperative medications to be given to Gary.

Fifth Hospital Day

Laboratory Results (Prior to the transplant surgery)

Red blood cell count		3.01 million per cu mm
Hemoglobin		9.3 gm/100 ml
Hematocrit		27.5%
Platelet count		178,000 per cu mm
White blood cell count		11,400 per cu mm
(differential)		
Segs	3%	
Lymphocytes	76%	
Monocytes	6%	
Eosinophils	7%	
Basophils	8%	
Cumulative lymphocyte count		833 per cu mm
Blood urea nitrogen		61 mg/100 ml
Creatinine		11.3 mg/100 ml

Gary slept well during the night. In the morning he weighed 102.5 pounds. When the nurse gave Gary his preoperative medications, he asked her why he had to have his side rails up and why he couldn't wear his class ring.

Study Questions

18. Compare the laboratory results on admission with those reported on Day 5. Identify what medications may have contributed to some of the changes.

19. What should the nurse respond to Gary's questions regarding the side rails and his class ring?

Gary Wong received his kidney transplant. His condition and his mother's condition were stable. Diuresis occurred within twenty minutes following the transplant.

Medical Orders

(1) Wear mask when entering room
(2) Flat in bed — do not turn patient — may raise left leg
(3) Weigh patient daily in A.M. before breakfast
(4) Record intake and output hourly (include an analysis of output: specific gravity, protein, sugar, blood, and ketones)
(5) Daily blood work: complete blood count, blood urea nitrogen, quantitative platelets, and absolute lymphocyte count
(6) 24-hour urine for creatinine clearance
(7) Gamma globulin 5 ml IM in each buttock now
(8) Prednisolone IM 40 mg stat., then 40 mg at 6:00 P.M., then 20 mg at midnight
(9) Starting tomorrow 6:00 A.M. dose: prednisolone 20 mg IM every 6 hours
(10) Diphenhydramine (Benadryl) 50 mg IM every 8 hours
(11) 1000 mg methylprednisolone sodium succinate (Solu-Medrol) in 150 ml 5% dextrose in water — to run over 1 hour

(12) Hydralazine hydrochloride (Apresoline) 10 mg s.c. if next diastolic pressure is above 110

(13) Furosemide (Lasix) 20 mg IV push now

(14) Vital signs hourly

(15) Meperidine hydrochloride (Demerol) 25 to 50 mg IM every 3 to 4 hours p.r.n. pain

(16) Trimethobenzamide (Tigan) 200 mg IM every 4 to 6 hours p.r.n. nausea and/or vomiting

(17) Intravenous fluids (alternate hourly 5% dextrose in lactated Ringer's solution and 5% dextrose with 0.45% sodium chloride solution) as follows:

- (a) For hourly output less than 25 ml, give 25 ml plus equivalent next hour
- (b) For hourly output between 25 and 50 ml, give 50 ml next hour
- (c) For hourly output between 51 and 100 ml, give equivalent volume next hour
- (d) For hourly output between 101 and 200 ml, give 100 ml or 80% of volume, whichever is greater
- (e) For hourly output between 201 and 400 ml, give 160 ml or 60% of volume, whichever is greater
- (f) For hourly output greater than 400 ml, call physician

Study Questions

20. What is the purpose of steroid therapy for Gary?

21. Discuss the pathophysiology of possible post-transplant complications and relate these to the drug therapy that has been ordered for Gary.

22. Describe the pharmacological action of gamma globulin and why it was administered to Gary.

23. Compare the action of gamma globulin to the preoperative immunosuppressive drugs that Gary received. Discuss the reason for administering 5 ml in each buttock.

24. As a result of the intravenous fluids and medications Gary is receiving, what can the nurse anticipate might happen to the serum sodium?

25. What effects do azathioprine and prednisolone have on Gary's platelet and leukocyte count?

26. Discuss the relationship between the order to wear masks and the medications that have been ordered for Gary.

27. What is the action of furosemide and why is it ordered for Gary?

28. What signs and/or symptoms might Gary show that would be indications of the effectiveness of furosemide? When will the nurse first be able to observe these?

29. What signs and/or symptoms should the nurse be alert to that would indicate toxic effects of azathioprine?

30. Discuss the relationship between the medications ordered for Gary and the checking of urine glucose content.

Sixth Hospital Day

Gary weighed 99 pounds. His hourly urine output ranged between 170 and 710 ml per hour; specific gravity ranged between 1.005 and 1.009. Gary's urine also indicated the presence of protein, glucose, blood, and ketones most of the day. Gary did show some signs of renal transplant rejection. This was evidenced in his diastolic blood pressure, which ran as high as 110 during that first postoperative day, and his temperature, which was increased to 101° F. during most of the day. Gary complained of some tenderness in the incisional site area as well as some nausea. He was effectively medicated with trimethobenzamide 200 mg IM for the nausea and meperidine 50 mg IM for the pain.

Study Questions

31. What nursing measures could be used to enhance the effects of the trimethobenzamide and the meperidine which Gary received on the first postoperative day?

32. Might the nausea that Gary experienced be related to any of the medications he received?

33. What assessments of Gary might have assisted the nurse in making the decision to give him meperidine 50 mg IM on the first postoperative day?

Seventh Hospital Day

Gary continued to experience rejection symptoms, and 150 rads of radiation to the kidney site was ordered for three days. Gary weighed 99 pounds and his urine output averaged 100 ml per hour. Specific gravity ranged between 1.012 and 1.024. Urine protein and glucose were decreasing, although blood in the urine ranged from a small amount to a large amount according to the tests being done by the staff nurses. Ketones were negative at that time.

Medical Orders

(1) Magaldrate (Riopan) 15 ml, and milk 15 ml every 2 hours while awake
(2) Clear liquids p.r.n., do not force
(3) Azathioprine (Imuran) 100 mg p.o. tonight
(4) Discontinue intravenous feedings at noon if intake p.o. is at least 600 ml
(5) Change diphenhydramine (Benadryl) and prednisolone to p.o. medications

Study Questions

34. Knowing the action of magaldrate, why was it ordered for Gary at this time? How does this differ from the preoperative orders for magaldrate?

35. Set up a schedule for the administration of magaldrate and milk for Gary.

36. In relation to corticosteroid therapy, what might the nurse anticipate in the future regarding Gary's weight?

Eighth through Sixteenth Hospital Days

Gary's hospitalization course continued with minimal problems. The protein, glucose, and blood that had previously been evident in Gary's urine were no longer present. Gary tolerated three radiation treatments well and incurred no problems other than slight nausea which was treated effectively with trimethobenzamide. Gary continued to lose weight and finally stabilized at 90 pounds. Although Gary's white blood count remained elevated, there was no significant increase in the blood count. Gary continued to have good renal functions, having a renal output of at least 1000 ml every 24 hours. His transplant functions were good. Although his daily azathioprine dosage was initially high, this was tapered down during this period of time.

Thirtieth Hospital Day

During the last two weeks of his hospitalization, Gary made progress. His laboratory tests indicated that his white blood cell count was still somewhat elevated but was beginning to return to normal. The red blood cell count, hematocrit, and hemoglobin levels returned to normal. Electrolyte and liver function studies were within normal limits.

At the time of discharge, Gary had a blood urea nitrogen of 29 mg/100 ml, a serum creatinine of 0.9 mg/100 ml, and a creatinine clearance of 66 ml uncorrected and 83 ml corrected.

<u>Discharge Orders</u>

(1) Azathioprine (Imuran) 75 mg p.o. daily
(2) Prednisolone 30 mg p.o. b.i.d.
(3) Diphenhydramine (Benadryl) 50 mg p.o. t.i.d.
(4) Multi-vitamins 1 capsule every day

Study Questions

37. Develop a teaching plan for Gary in relation to his medications and the occurrence of illnesses, such as flu or upper respiratory infections. Include a discussion of side effects in your plan.

38. What should Gary be taught about prednisolone?

39. Toxic symptoms of immunosuppressive therapy were not seen in Gary. Discuss what these symptoms are, and what changes in medications can occur when toxicity is present.

REFERENCES

Bois, M. S., et al.: Nursing care of patients having kidney transplant. Am. J. Nurs. 68:1677-1679, 1968.

Correa, A. L.: Current trends in diet and drug therapy for the dialysis patient. Nurs. Clin. N. Am. 10:469-479, 1975.

Martin, A.: Renal transplantation: surgical technique and complications. Am. J. Nurs. 68:1240-1241, 1968.

Schneider, W. J., and Boyce, B. A.: Complications of diuretic therapy. Am. J. Nurs. 68:1903-1907, 1968.

Shebelski, D.: Nursing patients who have renal hemotransplant. Am. J. Nurs. 66: 2425-2428, 1966.

7

THE PATIENT WITH CANCER OF THE PROSTATE

TEXTBOOKS SUGGESTED FOR THIS STUDY

Asperheim, M. K., and Eisenhauer, L. A.: The Pharmacologic Basis of Patient Care, ed. 2. W. B. Saunders Co., Philadelphia, 1973, Chapter 15.

Bergersen, B.: Pharmacology in Nursing, ed. 13. C. V. Mosby Co., St. Louis, 1976 Chapter 26

Brunner, L. S., and Suddarth, D.: Textbook of Medical Surgical Nursing, ed. 3. J. B. Lippincott Co., Philadelphia, 1975, Chapter 26.

Goodman, L., and Gilman, A. (eds.): The Pharmacological Basis of Therapeutics, ed. 5. Macmillan Co., New York, 1975, Chapters 15, 29, 38, 57, and 62.

Luckmann, J., and Sorensen, K.: Medical-Surgical Nursing — A Psychophysiologic Approach. W. B. Saunders Co., Philadelphia, 1974, Chapter 98.

Rodman, M. J., and Smith, D.: Pharmacology and Drug Therapy in Nursing. J. B. Lippincott Co., Philadelphia, 1974, Chapters 18, 36, 41, and 50.

Shafer, K. N., et al.: Medical Surgical Nursing, ed. 6. C. V. Mosby Co., St. Louis, 1975, Chapter 21.

PAST MEDICAL HISTORY

Mr. Sato, a busy 62-year-old business executive, has had intermittent minor back pain for the last 9 or ten years. An acute episode of this pain was treated effectively with pelvic traction five years ago. He was hospitalized three years ago for a small renal calculus which he expelled spontaneously. About one month ago, Mr. Sato's back pain returned and was accompanied by urinary urgency and frequency. The physician recommended a urologic workup and admitted him to the local hospital. Mr. Sato had no history of diabetes, hypertension, or heart trouble, and no known allergies.

PRESENT HOSPITAL ADMISSION

First Hospital Day

Mr. Sato's chief complaint upon admission was urinary frequency accompanied by a decreased urinary stream during the past month. Pain on urination was not present. In the admission interview, the nurse indicated that besides the lumbar pain Mr. Sato was also experiencing pain in both hips and thighs. Anorexia was present and had persisted for a couple of days prior to admission. Admitting vital signs were temperature 98.8° F., pulse 108, respirations 20, and blood pressure 170/80.

The admission physical examination showed a well developed and well nourished male in no acute distress. During the last month, Mr. Sato had lost six to eight pounds. His admission height was 65 inches and his weight was 165 pounds. Mr. Sato's abdomen was soft and his liver, spleen, and kidneys were not palpable. Extremities showed no edema, and neurological function was intact. Examination of the back revealed tenderness over the lumbar spine area. Mr. Sato's prostate gland was enlarged.

Mr. Sato's admitting diagnosis was prostatic hypertrophy.

Medical Orders

(1) Regular diet until 4:00 P.M. tonight
(2) Complete blood count in A.M.
(3) Blood urea nitrogen in A. M.
(4) Excretory urogram (IVP) in A.M.
(5) Chest x-ray in A.M.
(6) Acid phosphatase in A.M.
(7) Alkaline phosphatase in A.M.
(8) Cystoscopy and perineal needle biopsy of prostate in A.M.
(9) Acetaminophen with 30 mg of codeine phosphate (Tylenol #3) every 4 hours p.r.n. for back and/or leg pain
(10) Emulsified castor oil (Neoloid) 4 oz at 4:00 P.M. today
(11) Clear liquid dinner
(12) NPO after midnight
(13) Tap water enemas till clear in A.M.
(14) Diphenhydramine hydrochloride (Benadryl) 50 mg IV to be kept on the floor
(15) Electrocardiogram today
(16) Urinalysis today

Study Questions

1. Why have four oz of castor oil been ordered for Mr. Sato? Why has this been ordered prior to dinner rather than following dinner?

2. In what situations would castor oil be contraindicated?

3. How can the nurse evaluate the effectiveness of the castor oil administered to Mr. Sato?

In talking with the physician, the nurse learned that meglumine diatrizoate (Hypaque) is to be used as the dye during the excretory urogram. The physician asked the nurse to send the diphenhydramine with Mr. Sato when he leaves the floor for his excretory urogram because it is to be used during this test. During the rest of the evening, the focus of the nursing care for Mr. Sato was on preparing him for those tests and procedures which he was to have the next day.

Study Questions

4. The nurse explained to Mr. Sato that he would receive a radiopaque dye when

he had the excretory urogram. By what method of administration will this be given to Mr. Sato? Does this mean that Mr. Sato will be radioactive?

5. Mr. Sato asked what the purpose is of receiving this dye. What should the nurse respond?

6. Discuss the use of meglumine diatrizoate when a patient has known allergies.

7. What sensations may be felt by Mr. Sato when the contrast dye is administered? How long should Mr. Sato expect these sensations to last?

8. Why was diphenhydramine to be used during the excretory urogram?

Second Hospital Day

Mr. Sato tolerated his preparation for the procedures and tests well. During the night he slept at intervals, needing medication for back and leg pain only once. Mr. Sato continued to have difficulty with frequency and urgency, voiding in amounts of 75 to 100 ml approximately every two hours. Mr. Sato's electrocardiogram was within normal limits and his chest x-ray was essentially negative except for blastin changes of the ribs.

Laboratory Results

Complete blood count	
Red blood cell count	4.9 million per cu mm
Platelet count	149,000 per cu mm
White blood cell count	6,900 per cu mm
Hemoglobin	14.1 gm/100 ml
Hematocrit	40.7%
Blood urea nitrogen	19 mg/100 ml
Acid phosphatase	29 King-Armstrong units
Alkaline phosphatase	1740 Bodansky units
Blood chemistry	
Chloride	100 mEq/L
Bicarbonate	25 mEq/L
Potassium	3.7 mEq/L
Sodium	138 mEq/L

Mr. Sato was sent to the x-ray department for the excretory urogram which was to be followed by the cystoscopy. His vital signs preoperatively remained stable: temperature 98.8° F., pulse 108, respirations 20, and blood pressure 170/84.

Mr. Sato returned to his room following his excretory urogram and cystoscopy. Vital signs upon return to the floor were as follows: temperature 99.4° F., pulse 108, respirations 20, and blood pressure 160/74. Mr. Sato had a Foley catheter which was draining blood-tinged urine. He complained of some nausea and a headache. Results of the excretory urogram indicated a mild prostatic enlargement with trabeculation of the bladder. Initial results of the needle biopsy, carried out during the cystoscopy, showed adenocarcinoma of the prostate.

Medical Orders

(1) Regular diet
(2) Cephalexin monohydrate (Keflex) 250 mg p.o. every 6 hours
(3) Foley catheter to straight drainage
(4) Meperidine hydrochloride (Demerol) 50 - 75 mg every 4 hours p.r.n. for pain
(5) Bone scan tomorrow A.M.
(6) EKG tonight

Study Questions

9. Mr. Sato complained of nausea. Could this be related to any of the medications he has received? If so, which ones?

10. What is the action of cephalexin, and why was it ordered for Mr. Sato?

11. Cephalexin is effective against what type of organisms? Are there any indications that Mr. Sato has an infection?

13. What systemic effects should the nurse caring for Mr. Sato note as a result of cephalexin therapy?
What systemic effects should the nurse caring for Mr. Sato note as a result of cephalexin therapy?

14. Compare and contrast cephalothin and cephalexin. Why was cephalexin ordered for Mr. Sato rather than cephalothin?

15. Mr. Sato has an order for meperidine (Demerol) 50 - 75 mg every 4 hours p.r.n. for pain. Should this be given to Mr. Sato for his headache? What other nursing measures might be employed to decrease or eliminate Mr. Sato's headache?

Third Hospital Day

During Mr. Sato's third hospital day his nausea decreased and he was able to tolerate oral fluids. The previous 24-hour output totaled 720 ml and Mr. Sato's intake had been 1620 ml. His headache was gone and his back pain had been adequately relieved with meperidine 75 mg, which he had received twice. Results of the urinalysis were as follows:

Specific gravity	1.030
Albumin	faint trace
Sugar	negative

Fourth and Fifth Hospital Days

Mr. Sato continued to have intermittent back pain relieved effectively by meperidine. Anorexia began to improve and Mr. Sato was able to tolerate small feedings at meal time. The bone scan was completed, and interpretation confirmed the presence of widespread bone metastases. Palliative treatment was planned and included bilateral orchidectomy and estrogen therapy.

Medical Orders

(1) Soap suds enema tomorrow A.M.
(2) Shave pubis, scrotum and perineum
(3) Acetaminophen with 30 mg of codeine phosphate (Tylenol # 3) p.r.n. for pain
(4) Diethylstilbestrol 2 mg t.i.d. p.c.
(5) Discontinue meperidine hydrochloride (Demerol)
(6) NPO after midnight
(7) Preoperative medication to be given at 6:15 A.M.:
    Meperidine hydrochloride (Demerol) 50 mg IM
    Atropine sulfate 0.4 mg IM
    Hydroxyzine pamoate (Vistaril) 50 mg IM
(8) To surgery at 7:15 A.M.

Study Questions

16. What was the rationale for administering diethylstilbestrol to Mr. Sato preoperatively?

17. If Mr. Sato asks for something for pain at 1:00 A.M. after he is NPO, what would be the appropriate nursing action?

18. What is the action of the preoperative medications ordered for Mr. Sato? What effects will these medications have on Mr. Sato? What nursing actions will be necessary for Mr. Sato as a result of receiving these preoperative medications?

19. Discuss the preparation of the preoperative medication. Include factors influencing the number of injections needed and the methods for preparing and combining the medications.

Sixth Hospital Day

Mr. Sato tolerated the bilateral orchidectomy well. He was awake and his vital signs were stable when he returned from surgery. His scrotal dressing had been saturated once with serosanguineous drainage and had been reinforced. Ice had been applied to the incision and he was wearing a scrotal support. Mr. Sato had no scrotal discomfort although he did have some general complaints of not feeling well. His temperature at this time was 101.4° F.

Medical Orders

(1) Regular diet
(2) Foley catheter to straight drainage
(3) Meperidine hydrochloride (Demerol) 50 - 100 mg IM every 4 hours for pain
(4) Acetaminophen (Tylenol) 600 mg now, and then 300 mg t.i.d. for 2 days
(5) Acetaminophen with 30 mg of codeine phosphate (Tylenol #3) 1 tablet p.o. every 2 hours p.r.n. for pain
(6) Blood culture if oral temperature elevated above 102.5° F., or if patient has chills
(7) Complete blood count, platelets in A.M.

(8) Diethylstilbestrol 2 mg t.i.d.

Study Questions

20. Why was diethylstilbestrol ordered following Mr. Sato's orchidectomy?

21. What is the pharmacological action of diethylstilbestrol? What are its side effects? What nursing observations should be made in relationship to them?

22. Compare the action of the hormones produced by the testes with the action of estrogen.

23. What risks are associated with the diethylstilbestrol treatment Mr. Sato is receiving? How long will it be before the nurse should be observant for these risks in Mr. Sato?

Within five days following the initiation of the diethylstilbestrol therapy, Mr. Sato began to notice a decrease in leg pain. Mr. Sato experienced no additional problems and was discahrged on diethylstilbestrol 2 mg t.i.d. He is to return to the physician's office in one week.

Study Questions

24. What physical changes, including secondary sexual characteristics, might Mr. Sato experience as a result of diethylstilbestrol therapy? What preventive measures have been successful in controlling these changes?

25. How can the nurse help Mr. Sato to prepare for the possible changes he might experience as a result of diethylstilbestrol therapy?

26. One adverse side effect of long term diethylstilbestrol therapy is edema. Describe the physiological response to this medication that causes this effect.

27. Calcium levels are frequently elevated in patients receiving estrogen therapy. Why is this so?

28. Discuss the possible cardiovascular changes and related nursing care that might occur in relation to hypercalcemia.

29. What possible renal problems may be encountered by Mr. Sato as a result of being on estrogen therapy? What patient-teaching may be done by the nurse in relation to these problems?

30. Discuss the relationship of serum phosphatase levels to the dosage of diethylstilbestrol used to treat Mr. Sato.

REFERENCES

Donovan, M., and Pierce, S.: Cancer Care Nursing. Appleton Century-Crofts, New York, 1976, pp. 231-232.

Marino, E., and LeBlanc, D.: Cancer chemotherapy. Nursing '75, 5:22-23, 1975.

Rodman, M. J.: Anticancer chemotherapy: Part 1 — The kinds of drugs and what they do. R.N., 33:45-48+, 1972.

Rodman. M. J.: Anticancer chemotherapy: Part 2 — Against solid malignant tumors. R.N., 35:61+, 1972.

8

THE PATIENT WITH HYPERTENSION

TEXTBOOKS SUGGESTED FOR THIS STUDY

Asperheim, M. K., and Eisenhauer, L. A.: The Pharmacologic Basis of Patient Care. W. B. Saunders Co., Philadelphia, 1973, Chapters 13 and 19.

Beland, I., and Passos, J.: Clinical Nursing—Pathophysiological and Psychosocial Approaches, ed. 3. Macmillan Co., New York, 1975, Chapter 12.

Bergerson, B.: Pharmacology in Nursing, ed. 13. C. V. Mosby Co., St. Louis, 1976, Chapters 9 and 10.

Brunner, L. S., and Suddarth, D. S.: Textbook of Medical-Surgical Nursing, ed. 3. J. B. Lippincott Co., Philadelphia, 1975, Chapter 21.

Goodman, L., and Gilman, A. (eds.): The Pharmacological Basis of Therapeutics, ed. 5. Macmillan Co., New York, 1975, Chapters 12, 15, 26, 33, and 39.

Luckmann, J., and Sorensen, K.: Medical-Surgical Nursing—A Psychophysiologic Approach. W. B. Saunders Co., Philadelphia, 1974, Chapter 52.

Rodman, M. J., and Smith, D. W.: Pharmacology and Drug Therapy in Nursing. J. B. Lippincott, Philadelphia, 1974, Chapters 24, 25, and 26.

Sanderson, R.: The Cardiac Patient. W. B. Saunders Co., Philadelphia, 1972, Chapter 7.

Shafer, K., et al: Medical-Surgical Nursing, ed. 6. C. V. Mosby Co., St. Louis, 1975, Chapter 17.

PAST MEDICAL HISTORY

James Galloway, a 45-year-old man, was diagnosed as having moderate hypertension during a physical examination four years ago. At that time he stated that he did not feel well and suffered from mental and physical exhaustion. His blood pressure varied with the time of day, reaching its highest level (164/130) in the afternoon. He weighed 210 pounds and smoked one-and-one-half packages of cigarettes per day.

His physician prescribed hydrochlorothiazide (HydroDIURIL) 50 mg once a day and methyldopa (Aldomet) 500 mg twice a day. These medications resulted in his blood pressure dropping to 136/80 and remaining stable. He was given a 1500 Calorie diet with a no-added salt restriction and was advised to stop smoking. The nurse explained Mr. Galloway's medications, diet, and smoking restrictions to him and set up a schedule for checking his blood pressure and evaluating his program of treatment.

Immediately after the diagnosis of hypertension was made, Mr. Galloway followed the prescribed regimen. He lost 15 pounds, reduced his salt intake, and was only smoking about five cigarettes a day. Within a month he began to feel drowsy and experienced dizzy spells upon arising. He decided that his blood pressure must be too low and gradually stopped taking his pills. He began to feel better and neglected to keep scheduled appointments with his physician. As job and family pressures occurred, he started to smoke more heavily and his weight began to increase.

Study Questions

1. What type of medication is hydrochlorothiazide? What are its pharmacological actions? How does its site of action differ from furosemide and spironolactone?

2. The way in which diuretics control hypertension is not clearly understood. Discuss some of the theories related to their effectiveness.

3. Describe the type of nursing assessment that should be made before planning a teaching approach specific to Mr. Galloway's needs.

4. What should a patient be taught about the effects of hydrochlorothiazide? What aspects of patient teaching are needed to prevent adverse effects when a patient is taking thiazide diuretics at home?

5. Discuss the pharmacologic actions of spironolactone. Describe its effectiveness when given with hydrochlorothiazide.

6. Drugs affecting the sympathetic nervous system may be classified as:

   adrenergic drugs
   adrenergic blocking agents
   adrenergic neuron-blocking agents

   Discuss the action of each of these categories of drugs on the blood pressure. Mr. Galloway's prescribed medications belong to which categories?

7. Aldomet is an adrenergic neuron-blocking agent (adrenergic inhibiting drug). Discuss the present theories regarding its mechanisms of action. Name the other medications in this category and compare their action and side effects to spironolactone.

8. Mr. Galloway stopped taking his medication when he began having dizzy spells upon arising. Discuss the appropriateness of Mr. Galloway's response as it relates to the significance of his dizziness, lethargy, and drowsiness.

9. How might Mr. Galloway's lethargy be related to the administration of hydrochlorothiazide?

10. Mr. Galloway stopped seeing his physician once he began to feel better. Compare this pattern with that of most hypertensive patients and discuss ways by which this behavior might be averted.

11. What is the relationship between the use of drugs and the nonpharmacological treatment of Mr. Galloway's hypertension?

PRESENT HOSPITAL ADMISSION

First Hospital Day

8:30 P.M.—9:30 P.M. Mr. Galloway experiences the sudden onset of an occipital headache while watching television after dinner. At 8:30 P.M. it became so severe that his wife brought him to the emergency room of the local hospital. On admission, Mr. Galloway's vital signs were blood pressure 220/110, pulse 72 and regular, respirations 18, and temperature 97.8° F. orally. He was alert and did not have any visual disturbances, tinnitis, or parasthesias. His weight was 215 pounds. The following diagnoses were made:

(1) Hypertension
(2) Possible intracerebral pathology (bleeding thrombosis)

<u>Medical Orders</u>

(1) Bedrest
(2) Intravenous dextrose 5% in water at 5-10 drops per minute
(3) Diazoxide (Hyperstat I.V.) 300 mg IV bolus stat.
(4) Hydrochlorothiazide (HydroDIURIL) 50 mg p.o. now and b.i.d.
(5) Diazepam (Valium) 10 mg I.M. b.i.d. and h.s. Give first dose now.
(6) Meperidine hydrochloride (Demerol) 50 mg
Promethoazine hydrochloride (Phenergan) 25 mg — I.M. now and every 3 hours p.r.n. for severe headache
(7) Aspirin 600 mg
Codeine 30 mg — p.o. every 4 hours p.r.n. for mild to moderate headache
(8) Vital signs: every 10 minutes for 2 hours
every 30 minutes for 8 hours
If stable: every 1 hour for 2 hours
every 2 hours for 12 hours
(9) Neurological checks every 2 hours
(10) Diet 1200 Calories 2 gm sodium
(11) Intake and output
(12) Serum potassium, serum sodium, serum chloride, BUN stat. and in A.M.
(13) Blood glucose stat.
(14) Fasting blood glucose in A.M.
(15) Urine sugar and acetone q.i.d. Call physician if urine shows 2+ sugar.
(16) Weigh daily before breakfast

Study Questions

12. Describe how the nurse should administer the diazoxide. What problems may occur if it is administered into the tissues outside of the vein?

13. Both diazoxide and sodium nitroprusside are used for treating hypertensive crises. Compare these two medications including their onset of action, method of administration, and adverse effects.

14. Diazoxide is described as having a half-life of 28 $\pm$ 8.3 hours. What does this mean? What significance does this have when planning Mr. Galloway's nursing care?

15. Discuss the nursing observations that are related to the duration of action of diazoxide.

16. Discuss how the blood pressure should be taken for a patient in a hypertensive crisis. Include equipment used, position of patient and the personnel taking the blood pressure in your answer. How do the results obtained relate to the administration of the antihypertensive medications?

17. Blood sugar, urine sugar, and urine acetone tests were ordered even though Mr. Galloway had no history of diabetes. Why?

18. Compare the combined pharmacological effect of diazoxide and hydrochlorothiazide when given together to the effects of each drug given separately.

19. Discuss the pharmacological actions of diazepam. What nursing observations should be made when administering this medication?

20. Mr. Galloway received meperidine (Demerol) and promthazine hydrochloride (Phenergan) for a severe headache. Compare the combined pharmacological effect of these medications when given together to the effects of each drug when given separately. What effects on the blood presure, if any, may be expected from these medications?

21. What are the pharmacological effects of aspirin and codeine?

22. Discuss the nursing assessment that should be made by the nurse to differentiate between a severe and moderate headache.

9:30 P.M.—10:00 P.M. Following the administration of diazoxide, Mr. Galloway's blood pressure initially dropped to 132/56. It then began to rise and within 30 minutes it was 148/80. His headache was less severe and he was resting comfortably.

10:00 P.M.—12:00 P.M. Mr. Galloway's blood pressure was 150/90, pulse 84, and respirations 20. He was dozing between blood pressure readings and stated that he had only a mild headache.

Laboratory Results

Serum potassium	4.2 mEq/L
Serum sodium	142 mEq/L
Serum chloride	108 mEq/L
Blood urea nitrogen	18 mg/100 ml
Blood glucose	100 mg/100 ml

Second Hospital Day

12:00 P.M.—8:00 A.M. Mr. Galloway's blood pressure readings remained stable between 150/90 and 176/100. He complained of a moderate headache at 4:00 A.M. which was relieved by codeine and aspirin. Frequent urination and blood pressure readings during the night prevented prolonged periods of rest. Urine sugar and acetone tests were negative and his weight at 7:30 A.M. was 211 pounds.

8:00 A.M.—12:00 P.M. Mr. Galloway's headache did not return and he was feeling much better. He complained that he did not have enough food for breakfast and then did not finish what he had because he was not allowed to use salt. The physician visited and reevaluated Mr. Galloway's condition.

Medical Orders

(1) Take vital signs every 4 hours with sitting and standing blood pressures
(2) Bedrest with bathroom privileges
(3) Hydralazine (Apresoline) 25 mg p.o. b.i.d.
(4) Reduce diazepam (Valium) to 5 mg p.o. t.i.d.
(5) Serum potassium and serum sodium in A.M.

12:00 M.—4:00 P.M. Mr. Galloway's blood pressure remained stable between 140/80 and 150/90. He had a mild headache once during the day which was relieved by codeine and aspirin. Intracerebral pathology was thought unlikely when a lumbar puncture done at 12:00 P.M. was negative.

Laboratory Results

Serum potassium	4.0 mEq/L
Serum sodium	140 mEq/L
Fasting blood glucose	90 mg/100 ml

Study Questions

23. What plans for patient safety should be considered by the nurse caring for Mr. Galloway from 12:00 P.M. to 8:00 A.M. on the second hospital day? Consider the physiological response to diuretic and antihypertensive medications in your answer.

24. Accurate blood pressure readings are essential for patients receiving antihypertensive medications. Review the procedure for taking sitting and standing blood pressures. How can an error related to reading the sphygmomanometer be avoided?

25. What was Mr. Galloway's physiological response to diazoxide? Is this the normal response of patients in the accelerated phase of hypertension?

26. Hydralazine was ordered at 9:00 A.M. for Mr. Galloway. Compare the pharmacological action of this medication to the actions of adrenergic inhibitors.

27. What should the nurse tell Mr. Galloway about taking hydralazine?

Third Hospital Day

8:00 A.M.—4:00 P.M. Mr. Galloway slept most of the night. He complained of a mild headache at 8:00 A.M. which was relieved by codeine and aspirin. His blood pressure was 160/90 sitting and 145/100 standing; weight was 209 pounds.

Laboratory Results

Serum potassium	3.8 mEq/L
Serum sodium	139 mEq/L

Medical Orders

(1) Patient may use salt substitute
(2) Serum potassium now
(3) Discontinue neurological checks
(4) Discontinue intravenous
(5) Allow patient to be out of bed ad lib.

4:00 P.M.—12:00 P.M. Mr. Galloway complained of feeling dizzy when he was getting out of bed and told the nurse that this was how he felt at home when taking his medicine. He enjoyed his food more after he was given the salt substitute to use.

Study Questions

28. Relate the order for serum potassium levels to the pharmacological action of the drugs Mr. Galloway is receiving.

29. Discuss the relationship between Mr. Galloway's diagnosis of hypertension, his medication therapy with hydrochlorothiazide and hydralazine, and his dietary restriction.

30. Has Mr. Galloway's medication therapy been effective in treating his hypertension?

31. What substance is used as a salt substitute? Is it of any physiological value for Mr. Galloway? Consider his medication therapy in your answer.

32. What is the relationship between Mr. Galloway's weight loss, his diet, and his medication therapy?

Progress Report

Mr. Galloway remained in the hospital for one week. His headaches gradually disappeared and he began to feel well and rested. On the fourth hospital day his hydralazine was increased to 25 mg q.i.d. His standing and sitting blood pressure remained stable between 140/90 and 126/72. He had lost eight pounds and was getting used to his low-calorie diet. He asked the nurse how long he would have to take his medicine after his hypertension was cured.

Discharge Orders

(1) Hydralazine (Apresoline) 25 mg p.o. b.i.d.

(2) Hydrochlorothiazide (HydroDIURIL) 50 mg p.o. b.i.d.
(3) Instruct patient on a 1500 Calorie no-added-salt diet
(4) Teach patient to take blood pressure at home

Study Questions

33. How should the nurse answer Mr. Galloway's question about taking medication after his hypertension is cured?

34. In the past, Mr. Galloway stopped taking his medication because of adverse reactions. What nursing approaches can be used to prevent this from recurring?

35. Develop a teaching plan for Mr. Galloway that includes his dietary restrictions as well as medication therapy. Include the foods a patient taking hydrochlorothiazide should eat to prevent side effects.

36. What should Mr. Galloway be taught about the time of day his medications should be taken? Consider the pharmacological actions, their relationship to periods of sleep and wakefulness, and the circadian rhythm's effect on blood pressure.

REFERENCES

Aagard, G. N.: Treatment of hypertension, Am. J. Nurs., 73:621-623, 1973.

Conte, A., Brandzel, M., and Whitehead, S.: Group work with hypertensive patients, Am. J. Nurs., 74:910-912, 1974.

Finnerty, F. A.: Aggressive drug therapy in accelerated hypertension, Am. J. Nurs., 74:2176-2180, 1974.

Gluck, J.: Hypertension: caring for the patient who feels well, N '74, 4:74-76, 1974.

Griffith, E. W., and Madero, B.: Primary hypertension—patients' learning needs, Am. J. Nurs., 73:624-627, 1973.

Hussar, D.A.: Anti-hypertensive agents, N '74, 4:37-42, 1974.

Long, M., et al: Hypertension: what patients need to know, Am. J. Nurs., 76:765-770, 1976.

Robinson, A.M.: Detection and control of hypertension: challenge to all nurses, Am. J. Nurs., 76:778-780, 1976.

Rodman, M. J.: Drugs used in cardiovascular disease—treating hypertension, RN, 36: 41-54, 1973.

Shank, L. F., and Ludewig, J.: Hypertension, Nurs. Clin. N. Am., 9:677-692, 1974.

9

THE PATIENT WITH A CARDIAC ARREST

TEXTBOOKS SUGGESTED FOR THIS STUDY

Asperheim, M. K., and Eisenhauer, L. A.: The Pharmacologic Basis of Patient Care, ed. 2. W. B. Saunders Co., Philadelphia, 1973, Chapters 6, 12, 13, 15, and 17.

Bergersen, B.: Pharmacology in Nursing, ed. 13. C. V. Mosby Co., St. Louis, 1976, Chapters 9, 10, 11, and 16.

Brunner, L. S., and Suddarth, D.: Textbook of Medical Surgical Nursing, ed. 3. J. B. Lippincott Co., Philadelphia, 1975, Chapters 19 and 38.

Goodman, L., and Gilman, A. (eds.): The Pharmacological Basis of Therapeutics, ed. 5. Macmillan Co., New York, 1975, Chapters 12, 24, 32, 36, 37, and 71.

Luckmann, J., and Sorensen, K.: Medical-Surgical Nursing — A Psychophysiologic Approach. W. B. Saunders Co., Philadelphia, 1974, Chapter 50.

Rodman, M. J., and Smith, D.: Clinical Pharmacology in Nursing. J. B. Lippincott Co., Philadelphia, 1974, Chpaters 19, 23, and 29.

Shafer, K. N., et al.: Medical Surgical Nursing, ed. 6. C. V. Mosby Co., St. Louis, 1975, Chapter 17.

PAST MEDICAL HISTORY

John Brentwood, a 55-year-old policeman, has had a history of diabetes mellitus for two years. He was originally controlled on insulin and diet, and then treated successfully with oral hypoglycemic agents and diet. On the night of admission Mr. Brentwood had a sudden onset of overall discomfort with weakness, diaphoresis, and pain in his left arm. There was no dyspnea, chest pain, or severe chest discomfort. Nausea occurred and three episodes of vomiting produced partially digested food with no blood or coffee-ground material. He was taken to the emergency room of the local medical center by his wife.

PRESENT HOSPITAL ADMISSION

8:30 P.M.—8:45 P.M. Mr. Brentwood was admitted at 8:30 P.M., oriented, coherent, and cooperative. His weight was approximately 165 pounds. Although unable to localize any pain, he complained of feeling "lousy all over" and appeared restless and uncomfortable. An immediate chest examination revealed a very weak heart beat with abnormal extra-heart sounds. Because of the nature of the heart sounds an electrocardiogram was performed without awaiting further physical examination. The tracing revealed a normal sinus rhythm with occasional premature atrial contractions (PAC's) and changes compatible with the diagnosis of an acute inferior posterior myocardial infarction with lateral extension. As preparations were being made for transfer to the coronary unit, Mr. Brentwood had a cardiac arrest. Basic life support was begun immediately with the attending physician present and in charge of the situation.

8:45 P.M.—8:52 P.M. The cardiac arrest team initiated cardiopulmonary resuscitation, inserted a Foley catheter, started intravenous lines, and attached a cardiac monitor. Sodium bicarbonate was administered intravenously at 8:45 P.M. The monitor revealed ventricular fibrillation, and defibrillation with countershock was delivered at 8:48 P.M. At 8:49 P.M. Mr. Brentwood was moaning. Blood gases were drawn and sent to the laboratory and a nasogastric tube was inserted. Defibrillation was repeated, unsuccessfully, and cardiopulmonary resuscitation continued.

Study Questions

1. What is the action of sodium bicarbonate and why was it administered to Mr. Brentwood immediately? How does this method relate to the usual procedure in a cardiac arrest? Discuss the action of this drug as it relates to pathophysiological processes which occur during a cardiac arrest.

2. How does carbon dioxide elimination occur during Mr. Brentwood's cardiac arrest, and how does this relate to the administration of sodium bicarbonate?

3. Why was the intravenous route selected for administration of sodium bicarbonate? Discuss how this medication should be prepared and administered to Mr. Brentwood.

4. What relationship is there between the administration of sodium bicarbonate to Mr. Brentwood, the occurrence of ventricular fibrillation, and the use of the defibrillator?

5. How does Mr. Brentwood's history of diabetic control relate to his need for sodium bicarbonate during his cardiac arrest?

6. Discuss the need for arterial blood gas information in the evaluation of the medications being administered to Mr. Brentwood. Are medications such as sodium bicarbonate usually administered before these blood test samples are drawn? Why?

7. During a cardiac arrest, verbal orders are given for medications, and the form used to record the medications may serve as the verification of the orders. Discuss the legal implications of this method and compare it to the non-emergency situation.

8. Describe the relationship between the insertion of the Foley catheter and the administration of various drugs during a cardiac arrest.

8:52 P.M.—9:05 P.M. Mr. Brentwood continued to be maintained with cardiopulmonary resuscitation while the monitor revealed continued ventricular fibrillation. A 50 mg bolus of lidocaine was administered IV at 8:52 P.M. Defibrillation with countershock was delivered at 8:52 P.M. and 8:54 P.M. but was ineffective in converting the cardiac rhythm. The external chest compression continued and was effective in producing a good pulse. There was no pulse without compression. At 8:58 P.M., after Mr. Brentwood was intubated and a second dose of sodium bicarbonate was administered, there were still no pulses without chest compression. Adrenalin 1 mg was administered IV at 8:58 P.M. Defibrillation with countershock at 9:01 P.M. resulted in normal sinus rhythm. A 50 mg lidocaine bolus was administered IV at 9:02 P.M. for premature ventricular contractions; cardiopulmonary resuscitation continued.

Results of the 8:49 P.M. arterial blood gas study indicated the following:

pH	7.58
PaO_2	112 mm Hg
$PaCO_2$	29 mm Hg
Base excess	+6

CARDIAC ARREST MEDICATION RECORD FOR Mr. Brentwood

TIME PERIOD 8:45 P.M.—9:50 P.M.

Drugs and Intravenous Solutions	Route	Times	
Sodium bicarbonate 75 mEq	IV	8:45	8:58
37.5 mEq		9:09	9:22
		9:32	
Adrenalin 1 mg	IV	8:58	
Lidocaine 50 mg bolus	IV	8:52	9:02
Lidocaine 1 mg infusion	IV	9:06	
Regular Insulin 30 units	IV	9:05	
1000 ml 5% Glucose/Water started	IV	9:11	
Levarterenol 4 ml in 1000 ml 5% glucose in normal saline (4 ug/ml)	IV	9:14	
Diazepam 5 mg	IV	9:50	
Countershock		8:48	8:49
		8:52	8:54
		9:01	9:07
		9:12	

Study Questions

9. What is the action of lidocaine when used as an antiarrhythmic drug? How should the nurse evaluate the effectiveness of this medication?

10. Compare the action of lidocaine with the use of countershock in the treatment of ventricular arrhythmias.

11. What relationship is there between the untubation at 8:58 P.M. and the administration of a second dose of sodium bicarbonate?

12. What is the action of adrenalin and what results were expected when it was administered to Mr. Brentwood? What other drugs can be given which achieve effects

similar to adrenalin during a cardiac arrest?

13. Why is the intravenous route used to administer the adrenalin? By what other routes can it be given, in both life-threatening and non-life-threatening situations?

14. Relate Mr. Brentwood's blood gas results to drug therapy, other therapy, and Mr. Brentwood's pathophysiology. What additional medications can be anticipated?

9:05 P.M.—9:35 P.M. At 9:05 P.M. regular insulin 30 units was administered to Mr. Brentwood. At 9:06 P.M. Mr. Brentwood went into ventricular fibrillation again and a lidocaine intravenous infusion was begun. An unsuccessful defibrillation with countershock was carried out at 9:07 P.M. The lidocaine infusion was run at 20 drops per minute. Cardiopulmonary resuscitation continued. A third dose of sodium bicarbonate was administered at 9:09 P.M. and an infusion of glucose 5% in water was stated at 9:11 P.M. At 9:12 P.M. countershock was again administered with some initiation of response by Mr. Brentwood. An additional intravenous of normal saline with 2 ampules of levarterenol was begun immediately via an intravenous cutdown in the right arm. At 9:16 P.M. the electrocardiogram monitor demonstrated spontaneous normal sinus rhythm at a rate of 70/minute. Urine output was present but scant, and a blood pressure of 92 was present on palpation. The fourth dose of sodium bicarbonate was administered at 9:22 P.M. and the electrocardiogram continued to show normal sinus rhythm.

Blood pressure was audible at 128/80 and the levarterenol drip was continued at 24 drops/minute. In addition, the lidocaine continued to run at 20 drops/minute in the left arm. At 9:26 P.M. groaning by Mr. Brentwood was present and pulses were palpable. The levarterenol was running at 45 drops/minute at 9:32 P.M. with a blood pressure of 96/40 and pulse 68/minute. The last dose of sodium bicarbonate was administered.

Study Questions

15. Why was regular insulin administered to Mr. Brentwood?

16. Is regular insulin usually administered during a cardiac arrest?

17. Compare the administration of lidocaine in both intravenous bolus and intravenous solutions. What observations does the nurse need to carry out to determine the effectiveness of this medication?

9:35 P.M.—10:10 P.M. Mr. Brentwood began to have spontaneous movements in the lower extremities. His blood pressure at 9:40 P.M. was 204/130, pulse 80. The levarterenol was slowed from 40 drops/minute to 36 drops/minute. Mr. Brentwood began to have more movement in both upper and lower extremities. He sat up, rubbed his eyes, and said, "What are these?" as he pulled at his tubes. Diazepam 5 mg IV was ordered and given at 9:50 P.M. Mr. Brentwood seemed to calm down after this injection and blood gases were drawn and sent to the laboratory. At 10:06 P.M. levarterenol was continued at 50 drops/minute. The blood pressure was present at 110/90 and barely audible. Portable oxygen was connected and Mr. Brentwood was transferred to the coronary care unit.

18. Relate the need for a drug such as levarterenol to the pathophysiology of a cardiac arrest. What other drugs are used to treat this aspect of a cardiac arrest? Compare the advantages and disadvantages of these other drugs.

19. Explain the fluctuation of blood pressure in terms of the effectiveness of drug therapy. What can the nurse do to decrease this fluctuation?

20. What precautions are necessary to prevent adverse effects from the administration of levarterenol?

21. What is the action of diazepam and why is it indicated for the treatment of Mr. Brentwood?

22. Calcium chloride or calcium gluconate is frequently given in cardiac arrest. What is the intended action and how is it useful in an arrest situation?

23. Cerebral edema is a common complication of a cardiac arrest. What drugs commonly found on a cardiac arrest cart are used to treat this complication?

24. Discuss the occurrence of seizures during a cardiac arrest and the use of specific drugs for this complication.

REFERENCES

Betson, C.: Blood gases. Am. J. Nurs., 68:1010-1212, 1968.
Moyer, J. H., and Mills, L. C.: Vasopressor agents in shock. Am. J. Nurs., 75:620-625, 1975.
Standards for CPR and ECG. J.A.M.A., 227:835-867, 1974.
Ungvarski, P. J., Argondizzo, N. T., and Boos, P. K.: CPR — current practice revised. Am. J. Nurs., 75:236-247, 1975.

10

THE PATIENT WITH PULMONARY EMBOLISM

TEXTBOOKS SUGGESTED FOR THIS STUDY

Asperheim, M. K., and Eisenhauer, L. A.: The Pharmacologic Basis of Patient Care, ed. 2. W. B. Saunders Co., Philadelphia, 1973, Chapters 11, 14, and 17.
Beland, I., and Passos, J.: Clinical Nursing — Pathophysiological and Psychosocial Approaches, ed. 3. Macmillan Co., New York, 1975, Chapter 12.
Bergerson, B.: Pharmacology in Nursing, ed. 13. C. V. Mosby Co., St. Louis, 1976, Chapters 10 and 11.
Brunner, L. S., and Suddarth, D.: Textbook of Medical Surgical Nursing, ed. 3. J. B. Lippincott Co., Philadelphia, 1975, Chapters 15 and 19.
Goodman, L., and Gilman, A. (eds.): The Pharmacological Basis of Therapeutics, ed. 5. Macmillan Co., New York, 1975, Chapters 12, 15, 34, 49, and 65.
Luckmann, J., and Sorensen, K.: Medical-Surgical Nursing — A Psychophysiologic Approach. W. B. Saunders Co., Philadelphia, 1974, Chapter 65.
Rodman, M. J., and Smith, D.: Clinical Pharmacology in Nursing. J. B. Lippincott Co., Philadelphia, 1974, Chapters 13, 28, and 33.
Shafer, K., et al.: Medical Surgical Nursing, ed. 6. C. V. Mosby Co., St. Louis, 1975, Chapters 17 and 22.

PAST MEDICAL HISTORY

Mrs. Simms, a 57-year-old woman, was admitted for her seventh hospitalization. She was well until 13 years ago, when she had her first myocardial infarction at the age of 44 which was followed by a second one four years later. She has had other hospitalizations for severe angina. Two days prior to this admission, Mrs. Simms had crampy pains in both calves which lasted for one day. As the pain in her legs subsided, Mrs. Simms began to have severe left-sided chest pain which radiated down her left arm. Her stated height was 63 inches and weight, 135 pounds.

PRESENT HOSPITAL ADMISSION

First Hospital Day

7:00 A.M.—7:30 A.M. Mrs. Simms was admitted from the emergency room to the coronary care unit at 7:00 A.M., following a sleepness night of chest pain unrelieved by nitroglycerin (Nitrostat). On admission she had pleuritic left chest pain with left calf tenderness but no swelling or redness. An electrocardiogram was carried out immediately and showed no change from the ECG taken on her previous admission. The initial diagnostic impressions of the physician were:

(1) Possible myocardial infarction
(2) Possible pulmonary embolism
(3) Possible viral pleurisy

Medical Orders

(1) Meperidine hydrochloride (Demerol) 50-100 mg IM every 4 hours p.r.n. for pain
(2) Diazepam (Valium) 5 mg p.o. every 4 hours p.r.n. anxiety
(3) Acetaminophen (Tylenol) 650 mg p.o. every 4 hours p.r.n. for mild pain
(4) Nitroglycerin (Nitrostat) tabs 10 at bedside (0.4 mg)
(5) Electrocardiogram stat. and repeat in A.M.
(6) SGOT, CPK, and LDH stat. and repeat in A.M.
(7) Chest x-ray
(8) Ventilatory-perfusion lung scan

Study Questions

1. Identify the action of meperidine and describe how this action can be effective in relieving Mrs. Simms' chest pain.

2. Meperidine is considered a synthetic narcotic. What are the responsibilities of the nurse who administers this medication?

3. Why has the physician included a range of dosage for the meperidine order? What factors should the nurse take into account in determining how much meperidine to administer? Is this type of order legal in all states?

4. What signs and symptoms should the nurse look for to determine whether or not Mrs. Simms needs the diazepam?

5. What side effects of meperidine are potentially hazardous considering Mrs. Simms' possible diagnosis of cardiorespiratory problems? How should the nurse assess Mrs. Simms for the occurrence of these side effects?

6. What is the action of nitroglycerin?

7. What are the nursing responsibilities in carrying out the order for nitroglycerin tabs 10 at bedside?

7:30 A.M.—3:00 P.M. Mrs. Simms had been complaining of chest pain since admission. She was given meperidine 100 mg IM at 7:30 A.M. and again at 11:30 A.M. Mrs. Simms stated that the first pain medication given at 7:30 A.M. did not really relieve any pain. During this time the pain persisted, but she described it as being different from her earlier episodes of chest pain. The pain remained in the left side of her chest and shoulder but she described it as continual soreness rather than sharp and piercing. The pain increased on deep inspiration and upon movement. Mrs.

Simms' vital signs remained stable: blood pressure 108/80 to 114/80, pulse 80 to 84, respirations 20 to 22 and shallow. Her skin was warm and dry and no cyanosis was noted. Her husband was at her bedside as often as possible.

3:00 P.M.—7:30 P.M. Mrs. Simms began to get increasingly restless and began moaning. Meperidine 100 mg IM was administered at 3:30 P.M. along with diazepam 5 mg p.o. Following these medications, Mrs. Simms gradually stopped moaning, became drowsy, and was able to rest at intervals. She was able to take fluids for supper and got up to use the commode. At 7:30 P.M. another 50 mg of meperidine IM was administered following which Mrs. Simms said the pain was less.

Study Questions

8. What is the usual onset, peak, and duration of action for meperidine? How do these coincide with Mrs. Simms' response to the medication? When does she appear most comfortable?

9. How do you account for the change in the character of the pain following the second meperidine injection?

10. What are the factors in Mrs. Simms' situation which contribute to her pain response — pathophysiologic and psychosocial? What other nursing measures can be employed, besides administration of narcotics, in controlling Mrs. Simms' pain?

11. What is the action of diazepam when given with a narcotic and how does this differ from its action when given alone?

12. Describe the effects of the combined meperidine and diazepam administration on Mrs. Simms' signs and symptoms.

13. What signs and symptoms caused the nurse to decrease the meperidine to 50 mg at 7:30 P.M.?

14. What is the relationship of vital signs to potential side and toxic effects of meperidine?

7:30 P.M.—7:30 A.M. Mrs. Simms continued to have intermittent pain in her chest throughout the night but it was no longer described as radiating to the left shoulder or arm. She slept at intervals and complained of pain on movement and breathing. She got up to the commode once and her vital signs remained stable. Meperidine 50 mg was administered IM at 4- to 6-hour intervals and was effective in decreasing the pain. She complained of a cramp in her left leg once, which was relieved by pushing her heels against the bottom of the bed. At 7:30 A.M. Mrs. Simms said that she was tired of having the chest pain and hoped that it was not her heart. Diazepam 5 mg p.o. was administered following which Mrs. Simms ate a light breakfast.

Study Questions

15. Pain has both physiological and psychosocial causes. What actions of meperidine act to relieve each of these aspects?

16. Discuss communication approaches that the nurse can use when administering the meperidine to Mrs. Simms.

17. What is the significance of the leg cramping? Should the pain medications have been administered for this pain? Why?

Second Hospital Day

On the second hospital day, the reports on the electrocardiogram and serum enzymes indicated that no myocardial damage had occurred. The chest x-ray study indicated an infiltrate in the left base with pleural effusion, findings that could be secondary to either pneumonia or a pulmonary embolism with infarction. In the early afternoon the results of the ventilatory-perfusion lung scan revealed a well demarcated defect in the left middle lobe, characteristic of pulmonary embolism. The diagnosis of left pulmonary embolism was made.

Medical Orders

(1) Transfer out of coronary care to the intermediate medical care unit
(2) Oxycodone with aspirin, phenacetin, and caffeine (Percodan) 1 tablet p.o. every 3 hours p.r.n. pain
(3) Partial thromboplastin time stat. Then give heparin sodium (Panheprin) 8000 units IV followed by 4000 units every 4 hours IV
(4) Repeat partial thromboplastin time at 1:00 A.M. and notify the physician of results before giving the next heparin dose
(5) Prothrombin time stat. Then give warfarin sodium (Coumadin) 10 mg p.o. and repeat in A.M.
(6) Aluminum hydroxide, magnesium hydroxide, and simethione (Mylanta) 15-30 ml p.o. p.r.n. indigestion
(7) Prothrombin time in A.M.

Mrs. Simms was given the oxycodone for her pain and reported that it was much relieved. While soreness was still present, she felt she could take deep breaths more easily. Her spirits improved throughout the day. Vital signs remained stable.

Study Questions

18. Compare the action of oxycodone with the action of meperidine and discuss the differences that could occur in relieving Mrs. Simms' pain.

19. Explain how heparin acts in the body to prevent blood coagulation.

20. Why was the partial thromboplastin time done before and after the administration of heparin? Explain the difference in information about blood clotting derived from the partial thromboplastin time and the prothrombin time. How are these tests used to administer anticoagulant therapy? What are the nursing responsibilities related to obtaining these laboratory tests and administering the anticoagulant therapy?

21. Why is heparin administered intravenously? What other routes can be used?

22. Explain how warfarin acts as an anticoagulant.

23. Why were both heparin and warfarin ordered for Mrs. Simms?

24. What is the relationship between the actions of heparin and warfarin in the treatment of Mrs. Simms' pulmonary embolism?

25. What effects, if any, will heparin and warfarin have on the soreness and cramping in Mrs. Simms' leg? What other measures can be used to decrease these symptoms?

Second Hospital Night

At 1:00 A.M. the repeat partial thromboplastin time was drawn and the results of this and the previous partial thromboplastin time were as follows:

3:00 P.M. (2/15)	Initial partial thromboplastin time Patient 29.2 seconds Control 34.9 seconds
1:00 A.M. (2/16)	Second partial thromboplastin time Patient 100 seconds Control 38.2 seconds

Medical Orders

(1) Hold the 1:00 A.M. heparin dose
(2) Partial thromboplastin time stat. at 3:30 A.M. and call results to physician

At 3:30 A.M. the results of the partial thromboplastin time were as follows:

3:30 A.M. (2/16)	Third partial thromboplastin time Patient 40.5 seconds Control 38.0 seconds

These test results were followed with the heparin 4000 units administered at 5:00 A.M. During the night Mrs. Simms had intermittent chest pain which was relieved by oxycodone. When awakened for the blood tests at 1:00 A.M. and 3:30 A.M., Mrs. Simms complained of epigastric discomfort and received Mylanta 30 ml with relief of symptoms.

Study Questions

26. Why was the 1:00 A.M. dose of heparin held?

27. What specific antidote to heparin should the nurse have available for possible administration to Mrs. Simms?

28. What toxic effects of heparin would indicate the need for an antidote?

29. How can you account for the change in partial thromboplastin time from 1:00 A.M. to 3:30 A.M.? Is this change to be expected?

30. Why was heparin given again following the 3:30 A.M. partial thromboplastin time?

31. What is the action of Mylanta and how does it relieve the symptoms Mrs. Simms was experiencing?

32. What is the relationship between the pharmacological treatment of Mrs. Simms' pulmonary embolism and her symptoms of epigastric distress? Why is assessment and treatment of her gastric irritation important?

Third Hospital Day

Medical Orders

(1) Discontinue oxycodone with aspirin, phenacetin, and caffeine (Percodan)
(2) Acetaminophen (Tylenol) 650 mg every 4 hours for chest pain
(3) Daily prothrombin time starting today

Mrs. Simms continued to have less chest pain which was relieved by the acetaminophen. Her vital signs remained stable and her appetite was improving. An episode of gastric distress followed a visit by her husband. When he left, Mrs. Simms asked for the Mylanta stating that an argument with her husband had upset her. She was able to get up to the commode without assistance and could move in bed with much less distress.

Study Questions

33. Considering the chemical composition of oxycodone, why did the physician change the order from oxycodone to acetaminophen?

34. How does the action of Mylanta relate to the relief of Mrs. Simms' discomfort following an argument with her husband?

35. How should the nurse assess Mrs. Simms for the possible side effects of Mylanta?

36. What does the prothrombin time measure and why is it ordered on a daily basis for Mrs. Simms?

37. What is the relationship between the results of the daily prothrombin time and the administration of warfarin?

Medical Orders

(1) Daily partial thromboplastin time starting 2/17 A.M.
(2) Heparin sodium (Panheprin) 4000 units IV every 4 hours

HEPARIN RECORD

Date	Time	Partial Thromboplastin Time	Heparin Dose	Time
2/15	3:00 P.M.	Patient 29.2 sec		
		Control 34.9 sec	8000 U	6:00 P.M.
			4000 U	9:30 P.M.
2/16	1:00 A.M.	Patient 100 sec		
		Control 38.2 sec	4000 U HOLD	1:00 A.M.
	3:30 A.M.	Patient 40.5 sec		
		Control 38.0 sec	4000 U	5:00 A.M.
	9:00 A.M.	Patient 51.2 sec		
		Control 36.6 sec	4000 U	10:00 A.M.
	1:00 P.M.	Patient 57.7 sec		
		Control 37.6 sec	5000 U	2:00 P.M.
	6:00 P.M.	Patient 78.6 sec		
		Control 39.5 sec	4000 U	7:00 P.M.
	10:00 P.M.	Patient 75.4 sec		
		Control 38.0 sec	4000 U	11:30 P.M.
2/17	3:00 A.M.	Patient 55.9 sec		
		Control 37.9 sec	4000 U	4:00 A.M.
2/17	7:00 A.M.	Patient 60.3 sec		
		Control 36.7 sec	4000 U	8:00 A.M.
			4000 U	12:00 P.M.
			4000 U	4:00 P.M.
			4000 U	8:00 P.M.
			4000 U	12:00 A.M.
			4000 U	4:00 A.M.
2/18	7:00 A.M.	Patient 59.7 sec		
		Control 38.2 sec	4000 U	8:00 A.M.
			4000 U	12:00 P.M.

Study Questions

38. What advantages can you see from the use of a record such as the above for the administration of anticoagulant therapy?

39. Why was the dosage of heparin 4000 units held at 1:00 A.M. on 2/16?

40. Why was the dosage of heparin increased to 5000 units at 2:00 P.M. on 2/16?

41. Why did the physician decrease the partial thromboplastin time from every four hours to daily on 2/17?

42. Why was the heparin discontinued on 2/18?

WARFARIN RECORD

Date	Prothrombin	Warfarin Dose	Time
2/16	100.0%	10.0 mg	9:30 A.M.
2/17	31.5%	5.0 mg	1:10 P.M.
2/18	24.0%	5.0 mg	2:45 P.M.
2/19	31.0%	7.5 mg	2:35 P.M.
2/20	25.5%	5.0 mg	2:45 P.M.
2/21	22.0%	5.0 mg	2:45 P.M.
2/22	25.0%	5.0 mg	2:00 P.M.
2/23	22.0%	5.0 mg	1:00 P.M.
2/24	16.5%	0.0	
2/25	32.0%	5.0 mg	3:00 P.M.
2/26	38.0%	10.0 mg	11:55 A.M.
2/27	19.0%	5.0 mg	12:00 P.M.
2/28	16.5%	2.5 mg	10:45 A.M.

Study Questions

43. Why was the warfarin dosage increased on 2/19 to 7.5 mg?

44. Why was no warfarin given on 2/24?

45. Why was the dosage of warfarin decreased on 2/28?

46. What is the specific antidote for warfarin? Identify the various trade names and doses used.

Summary of Hospitalization from 3rd to 16th Hospital Days

Mrs. Simms continued to improve, although she continued to experience some chest pain with deep breathing. The tenderness in her calf was minimal and her chest clear to auscultation. She took nitroglycerin occasionally for chest pain with some relief. A repeat chest x-ray study on the 12th hospital day showed clearing of the left lower lobe infiltrate. A repeat lung scan on the same day showed improvement, with specific results showing minimal decrease in ventilation at the left lung base and slight residual perfusion decrease with no new areas of involvement. Discharge on the 14th hospital day was postponed because of the prothrombin time on that day. On the 16th hospital day Mrs. Simms was discharged.

Discharge Orders

(1) Warfarin sodium (Coumadin) 2.5 mg # 100, 1 and 2 tablets p.o. on alternate days
(2) Isosorbide dinitrate (Isordil) 10 mg # 100, 1 p.o. q.i.d.
(3) Visiting nurse follow-up for one visit
(4) Come in to the clinic for a prothrombin time one week from today. Call M.D. for results

Study Questions

47. What change in prothrombin time on 2/27 prompted the physician to cancel Mrs. Simms' discharge?

48. Explain the meaning of the discharge order for warfarin and discuss how Mrs. Simms should be instructed in taking this medication.

49. What side and toxic effects of warfarin should be included in giving discharge instruction to Mrs. Simms?

50. Describe the relationship between warfarin administration and the use of other medications, especially acetylsalicylic acid. What aspects of this relationship would you include in Mrs. Simms' medication instruction in order to prevent toxicity?

51. What information should the staff nurse discharging Mrs. Simms give to the visiting nurse who will do the follow-up visit at Mrs. Simms' home?

52. What aspects of anticoagulant therapy should the visiting nurse reinforce with Mrs. Simms?

53. What type of medication is isosorbide dinitrate? Why has it been ordered for Mrs. Simms?

Follow-Up Clinic Visit

Mrs. Simms arrived promptly at the clinic for her prothrombin time one week after discharge. She seemed at ease and stated that she had been taking her pills regularly and showed the nurse the daily record she was keeping. During the conversation Mrs. Simms mentioned that her sister had taken this medication several years previously and began to have bloody urine. She also mentioned that she was due for her annual gynecologic examination and her annual dental check-up at the clinic and would make the appointments while she was there. The nurse explained the relationship between warfarin therapy and bloody urine and emphasized the need to inform the gynecologist and dentist about her anticoagulant therapy. The nurse reminded Mrs. Simms to call the physician's office that afternoon for the results of the test and to return in a week for another prothrombin time.

Study Questions

54. Why are weekly prothrombin tests being done on Mrs. Simms? When and why will the frequency of these tests decrease or increase?

55. What should be included in the explanation of the relationship between administration of warfarin and the occurrence of bloody urine?

56. Why is it necessary to inform the gynecologist and the dentist that Mrs. Simms is on anticoagulant therapy?

REFERENCES

Beshore, J.: How to prevent — and if necessary treat — emboli. R.N. 38:29-35, 1975.

Dipalma, J.R.: Precautions with the anticoagulants. R.N. 34:57-66, 1971.

Fitzmarice, J. B., and Sasahara, A. A.: Current concepts of pulmonary embolism: implications for nursing practice. Heart Lung 3:209-218, 1974.

Hussar, D. A.: Cardiac drugs today — anticoagulants. Nursing '73, 4:11-15, 1973.

Kratz, A. M., and Kratz, J. L.: Cardiac drugs today — Vasodilators. Nursing '73, 5:33-37, 1973.

Leary, J. A., Vessels, D. M., and Yeaw, E. M.: Self-administered medications. Am. J. Nurs. 71:1193-1194, 1971.

Mayer, G. G.: Disseminated intravascular coagulation. Am. J. Nurs. 73:2067-2069, 1973.

Rodman, M. J.: Drugs that affect blood coagulation. R. N. Part 1 — 32:59-62, June, 1969. Part 2 — 32:59-62, July, 1969.

Sasahara, A., and Foster, V.: Pulmonary embolism: recognition and treatment. Am. J. Nurs. 67:1634-1641, 1967.

Shapiro, R.M.: Anticoagulant therapy. Am. J. Nurs. 74:439-443 , 1974.

Wessler, S., and Alexander, B.: A Guide to anticoagulant therapy. Am. Heart Assn., 1970.

Wyper, M.: Pulmonary embolism: fighting the silent killer. Nursing '75, 10:30-38 1975.

11

THE PATIENT WITH LEUKEMIA

TEXTBOOKS SUGGESTED FOR THIS STUDY

Asperheim, M. K., and Eisenhauer, L. A.: The Pharmacologic Basis of Patient Care, ed. 2. W. B. Saunders Co., Philadelphia, 1973, Chapters 15 and 20.

Bergersen, B.: Pharmacology in Nursing, ed. 13. C. V. Mosby Co., St. Louis, 1976, Chapters 24 and 25.

Brunner, L. S., and Suddarth, D.: Textbook of Medical Surgical Nursing, ed. 3. J. B. Lippincott Co., Philadelphia, 1975, Chapter 12.

Goodman, L., and Gilman, A. (eds.): The Pharmacological Basis of Therapeutics, ed. 5. Macmillan Co., New York, 1975, Chapters 15, 48, and 62.

Luckmann, J., and Sorensen, K.: Medical-Surgical Nursing — A Psychophysiologic Approach. W. B. Saunders Co., Philadelphia, 1974, Chapters 33, 34, and 35.

Rodman, M. J., and Smith, D.: Clinical Pharmacology in Nursing. J. B. Lippincott Co., Philadelphia, 1974, Chapters 17 and 48.

Shafer, K. N., et al.: Medical Surgical Nursing, ed. 6. C. V. Mosby Co., St. Louis, 1975, Chapter 15.

PAST MEDICAL HISTORY

Mrs. Lee, a 35-year-old career woman, was admitted to the hospital for removal of rectal polyps. Mrs. Lee had experienced no serious illnesses prior to her hospitalization. Childhood diseases included chicken pox at age 5, and measles and mumps at age 7. At age 13 she was hospitalized for an appendectomy. Recent history revealed one or two uncomplicated upper respiratory infections each year. She had no known heart trouble, hypertension, diabetes, or tuberculosis.

PRESENT HOSPITAL ADMISSION

First Hospital Day

The admission history and physical revealed that Mrs. Lee had experienced dizziness and easy fatigability of several weeks' duration. The dizziness occurred primarily upon exertion. She had been more tired than usual even though her daily routine had not changed. Her skin was warm and dry with no evidence of bruising or petechia. She had no bone tenderness, no hepatomegaly, and no splenomegaly. There was no evidence of lymphadenopathy. Admission vital signs included temperature

99.0° F., pulse 86, respirations 14, and blood pressure 110/76. The physical examination further revealed no evidence of present upper respiratory involvement, and Mrs. Lee's chest was clear to auscultation and palpation.

Medical Orders

(1) Soft diet
(2) Bathroom privileges
(3) Weigh daily and record
(4) Routine complete blood count
(5) Urinalysis
(6) Chest x-ray
(7) Diazepam (Valium) 5 mg p.o. t.i.d.
(8) Chloral hydrate (Noctec) 1 gm p.o. p.r.n. for sleep h.s.
(9) Abdominal prep
(10) NPO after midnight
(11) Preoperative medication: on call, IM
    Meperidine (Demerol) 50 mg
    Atropine sulfate 0.4 mg
    Hydroxyzine (Vistaril) 50 mg

Second Hospital Day

Laboratory Results

Urinalysis		normal
Chest x-ray		normal
Complete blood count		
Red blood cell count		2.48 million per cu mm
Platelet count		142,000 per cu mm
White blood cell count		2,000 per cu mm
(differential)		
Blasts	6%	
Stabs	1%	
Segs	22%	
Lymphocytes	64%	
Monocytes	7%	

Based on the results of her laboratory tests, only the visible rectal polyp was removed under local anesthesia. Mrs. Lee's vital signs were stable and she was afebrile following the removal of the polyp. She continued to experience some dizziness but had no other complaints.

Medical Orders

(1) Daily blood work
(2) Acetaminophen with 30 mg of codeine phosphate (Tylenol # 3) p.o. every 3 to 4 hours p.r.n. for pain

Study Questions

1. Why was chloral hydrate ordered for Mrs. Lee? What is its drug classification and how does it act? Identify other medications that are in the same drug classification as chloral hydrate.

2. Differentiate between salicylates and Tylenol # 3. Why has Tylenol # 3 been ordered for Mrs. Lee rather than one of the salicylates? Include an evaluation of Mrs. Lee's laboratory results in your answer.

3. What nursing observations should Mrs. Lee be watched for considering the medications she is receiving and her laboratory results? What nursing precautions can be taken in relation to this?

Third Hospital Day

The pathology report on the rectal polyp indicated no evidence of cancer cells. Mrs. Lee's condition continued to be stable. Daily white blood cell counts continued to be low normal and a bone marrow test was scheduled.

Study Questions

4. Mrs. Lee has now been on diazepam for two days. How should the nurse assess the effectiveness or ineffectiveness of the medication?

5. Mrs. Lee was admitted with complaints of dizziness and fatigue. Will these symptoms interfere with the nurse's evaluation of the effectiveness of the diazepam?

Fourth Hospital Day

The bone marrow aspiration, done at 10:00 A.M., was obtained from the sternum. Results showed a 50 per cent infiltration by lymphoblastic cells with a reduction of myelocytic cells. Mrs. Lee's case was presented at the tumor conference and a diagnosis of acute monocytic leukemia, aleukemic, was made.

Medical Orders

(1) Continue routine complete blood count daily
(2) Continue platelet count daily
(3) Magnesium trisilicate (Gelusil) 30 ml q.i.d.
(4) Chemotherapy orders
 (a) Vincristine sulfate (Oncovin) 2 mg IV on day 1, to be given by chemotherapy nurse
 (b) Prednisone (Meticorten) 25 mg q.i.d. orally for 5 days, to be given by floor nurse and recorded on chemotherapy sheet
 (c) Cytarabine (Cytosar) 180 mg IV infusion for 5 days in 1 L of 5% dextrose in distilled water, to be mixed and started by chemotherapy nurse
 (d) Cyclophosphamide (Cytoxan) 180 mg IV daily for 5 days, given as a single rapid injection every day to be given by chemotherapy nurse

Seventh Hospital Day

Mrs. Lee continued to be tired, often taking both morning and afternoon naps. She had no evidence of abnormal bleeding. Following the removal of the rectal polyp, Mrs. Lee requested the Tylenol # 3 on two occasions within the first 24 hours following surgery. The first course of chemotherapy was begun. The intravenous infusion was started by the chemotherapy nurse who also administered the vincristine and cyclophosphamide. The prednisone was administered by Mrs. Lee's team leader.

Study Questions

6. Discuss the advantages and disadvantages of multiple drugs for treatment of Mrs. Lee's leukemia.

7. Vincristine is a plant extract. What is its action? Include its effect on cell growth in your answer.

8. What is the relationship of vincristine to the other antineoplastic agents ordered for Mrs. Lee?

9. Discuss the rationale for intravenous infusion of vincristine. What other routes are used to administer this medication? In what other neoplastic diseases would these alternative routes be used?

10. If the infusion of vincristine infiltrates, what should the nurse do? What effects would an infiltration have on Mrs. Lee? What nursing observations are important in relation to infusions?

11. What signs and symptoms during infusion would indicate the need to discontinue Mrs. Lee's infusion immediately?

12. Prednisone is a steroid. What are the pharmacological actions of this group of medications?

13. Compare the action of prednisone with other steroid preparations.

14. Discuss the current theories related to the use of prednisone in the treatment of acute monocytic leukemia.

15. What side and/or toxic effects can be anticipated with the administration of steroids to Mrs. Lee?

16. Cytarabine has been ordered to be given by continuous infusion. What nursing responsibilities relate directly to this method of medication administration? What is the action of cytarabine? Include its effect on cell growth in your answer.

17. Since infection causes approximately 25 per cent of the deaths of patients with acute leukemia, what principles of asepsis should be used in administering intravenous medications to Mrs. Lee?

18. For how many hours should the infusion of cytarabine be administered?

19. Discuss the meaning of the order, "Cytarabine 180 mg IV infusion for 5 days..." Include the frequency and duration of each dose and the reason for these interpretations.

20. What problems might Mrs. Lee experience with the infusion of cytarabine that would directly relate to discontinuing the infusion?

21. Chemotherapy may be administered by local perfusion. Discuss this method and its use. Would this type of administration be used in the case of Mrs. Lee? Why?

22. Compare the use of antimetabolites and alkylating agents in the treatment of leukemia. Give an example of an antimetabolite and an alkylating agent from Mrs. Lee's drug list.

23. Compare the side and toxic effects of antimetabolites and alkylating agents to steroids and plant extracts. List the problems related to the side effects and toxic effects.

24. Discuss the responsibilities of a chemotherapy nurse in relation to the administration of medications to Mrs. Lee and similar patients.

Eighth Hospital Day

Eight hours after the initiation of the chemotherapy, Mrs. Lee experienced nausea and vomited a large amount of undigested food. The physician was notified and Mrs. Lee was given a stat. dose of benzquinamide hydrochloride (Emete-con) IM which gave her some relief from the nausea.

Laboratory Results

White blood cell count	2200 per cu mm
Red blood cell count	2.55 million per cu mm
Hemoglobin	9.6 gm/100 ml
Hematocrit	28.7%
Platelet count	120,000 per cu mm

Mrs. Lee's vital signs were stable with the exception of an elevated temperature of 102° F. Her only other complaints were of continued dizziness and tiredness. Mrs. Lee was placed in reverse isolation as a precautionary measure.

Medical Orders

(1) Benzquinamide hydrochloride (Emete-con) 50 mg IMq4h p.r.n. nausea/vomiting
(2) Magnesium hydroxide (Milk of Magnesia) 30 ml p.r.n. constipation

Study Questions

25. Describe the side and toxic effects experienced by Mrs. Lee on the eighth

hospital day. Relate these signs to specific drug action.

26. What nursing measures will minimize side and/or toxic effects? Discuss these nursing measures in relation to each sign or symptom.

27. Discuss the relationship between the placement of Mrs. Lee in reverse isolation and the effect the medications are having on her body. How should this be explained to Mrs. Lee?

28. How are medications administered to someone who is in reverse isolation?

29. What is the action of benzquinamide and why was it given to Mrs. Lee?

30. How should the nurse evaluate the effectiveness of benzquinamide?

Progress Report

Mrs. Lee continued to have some nausea but otherwise was asymptomatic, and the remainder of the chemotherapy course was completed. Following the completion of the course in chemotherapy, Mrs. Lee's nausea subsided. She remained in the hospital for two more days and was then discharged. At that time another bone marrow aspiration was done. This showed a normoplastic marrow with less than 10 per cent leukemia cells which were identified as monoblast. Blood work indicated a white blood count of 2400.

It was planned to evaluate Mrs. Lee in five days, after which a decision regarding further courses of chemotherapy would be made. No discharge medications were sent home with Mrs. Lee.

Study Questions

31. Why were Mrs. Lee's steroids abruptly discontinued rather than slowly decreased?

32. What indications will the physician use in determining the effectiveness of Mrs. Lee's first course of chemotherapy?

33. List chemotherapy side effects that Mrs. Lee Might experience after her discharge from the hospital. What precautionary measures should be discussed prior to discharge?

34. Considering the fact that Mrs. Lee's white blood count was 2400 at the time of discharge, what teaching should be done by the nurse?

REFERENCES

Bloomfield, K. J.: Johnny is my most difficult. . .and dearest. . .patient. Nursing '74, 4:68-70, 1974.

Dreizen, S., Bodey, G., Rodrigues, V., and McCredie, K.: Cutaneous complications of cancer chemotherapy. Post-grad. Med. 58:150-158, 1975.

Dreizen, S., Bodey, G., and Rodrigues, V.: Oral complications of chemotherapy. Post-grad. Med. 58:175-182, 1975.

Golden, S.: Cancer chemotherapy and management of patient problems. Nurs. Forum 14:278-303, 1975.
Marino, E., and LeBlanc, D. H.: Cancer chemotherapy. Nursing '75, 5:22-23, 1975.
Rodman, M. J.: Anticancer chemotherapy: Part 1 — the kinds of drugs and what they do. R.N. 35:45-48+, 1972.
Rodman, M. J.: Anticancer chemotherapy: Part 3 — against the leukemias and lymphomas. R. N. 35:49-50+, 1972.
Schumann, D., and Patterson, P. C.: The adult with acute leukemia. Nurs. Clin. N.Am. 7:743-761, 1972.

12

THE PATIENT WITH A SEIZURE DISORDER

TEXTBOOKS SUGGESTED FOR THIS STUDY

Asperheim, M. K., and Eisenhauer, L. A.: The Pharmacologic Basis of Patient Care, ed. 2. W. B. Saunders Co., Philadelphia, 1973, Chapter 11.

Bergersen, B.: Pharmacology in Nursing, ed. 13. C. V. Mosby Co., St. Louis, 1976, Chapter 11.

Brunner, L. S., and Suddarth, D.: Textbook of Medical-Surgical Nursing, ed. 3. J.B. Lippincott Co., Philadelphia, 1975, Chapter 35.

Goodman, L., and Gilman, A. (eds.): The Pharmacological Basis of Therapeutics, ed. 5. Macmillan Co., New York, 1975, Chapters 13, 15, 36, 62, 69, 70, and 73.

Luckmann, J., and Sorensen, K.: Medical-Surgical Nursing — A Psychophysiologic Approach. W. B. Saunders Co., Philadelphia, 1974, Chapter 39.

Rodman, M. J., and Smith, D.: Clinical Pharmacology in Nursing. J. B. Lippincott Co., Philadelphia, 1974, Chapter 12.

Shafer, K. N., et al.: Medical-Surgical Nursing, ed. 6. C. V. Mosby Co., St. Louis, 1975, Chapter 32.

PRESENT HOSPITAL ADMISSION

Mrs. Cooper, a 52-year-old housewife, had a left radical mastectomy seven years ago as a consquence of adenocarcinoma. She had metastatic lesions of the spine and had been treated on an outpatient basis with cyclophosphamide (Cytoxan) and fluoxymesterone (Halotestin) prior to admission. Mrs. Cooper had moderate to severe back pain in the past year for which she took a compound containing oxycodone with aspirin, phenacetin, and caffeine (Percodan) 1 tablet every 4 hours p.r.n.

First Hospital Day

On the day prior to hospitalization Mrs. Cooper began having left-sided clonic twitches which occasionally occurred bilaterally. She was awake and responsive but was unable to care for herself and was incontinent with the onset of seizures. She was also noted to be somewhat confused. Following arrangements made by the physician, Mr. Cooper took his wife to the hospital where she was admitted directly to the neurological unit. Her admitting diagnosis was "seizure disorder secondary to central nervous system metastasis." Cyclophosphamide and fluoxymesterone were discontinued.

Medical Orders

(1) Diphenylhydantoin (Dilantin) 100 mg IV stat. (given at 2:30 P.M.)
(2) Full liquid diet as tolerated p.o.
(3) Intravenous fluids: 5% dextrose in water with potassium chloride 15 mEq and vitamin B and C (Berocca C) 1 ampule alternating with 5% dextrose in 0.45% saline at 100 ml/hour
(4) Oxycodone with aspirin, phenacetin, and caffeine (Percodan) 1 tablet p.o. every 3 to 4 hours p.r.n. for pain
(5) Dexamethasone (Decadron) 8 mg IV stat. and 2 mg t.i.d. p.o.
(6) Hemoglobin, hematocrit and white blood count
(7) Serum sodium, potassium, chlorides, carbon dioxide, glucose, urea nitrogen, calcium, phosphate, uric acid, cholesterol, and LDH

Study Questions

1. Review the action of cyclophosphamide and fluoxymesterone when used for treatment of adenocarcinoma of the breast.

2. What assessment is necessary to determine adverse effects of cyclophosphamide and fluoxymesterone? What kind of findings would prompt institution of protective measures for Mrs. Cooper?

3. What was the reason for the administration of dexamethasone to Mrs. Cooper? What observations are necessary to determine effectiveness of this drug?

4. Compare Mrs. Cooper's drug therapy for her seizure disorder with that of a patient who has epilepsy.

5. Why is diphenylhydantoin ordered stat.? Discuss the preparation and administration of this order.

6. What is the action of diphenylhydantoin at the cellular level? Relate this action to the electrical activity associated with a seizure.

7. How does diphenylhydantoin compare in action to phenobarbital in the treatment of seizures?

8. How long will the 100 mg of diphenylhydantoin administered intravenously be effective?

Second Hospital Day

Mrs. Cooper was alert and oriented. No seizures were reported until 9:00 P.M. when she began having tremors of her left arm, extending to her left leg.

Medical Orders

(1) Diphenylhydantoin 100 mg IM stat. (given at 9:15 P.M.)
(2) Diphenylhydantoin 300 mg daily p.o.
(3) Diazepam (Valium) 10 mg every 4 hours p.o.

Laboratory Results

Serum Electrolytes	
Sodium	130 mEq/L
Potassium	4.3 mEq/L
Chloride	105 mEq/L
Carbon Dioxide	28 mEq/L
Calcium	9.5 mEq/L
Phosphate	3.5 mEq/L
White blood cells	6350 per cu mm
Blood glucose	150 mg/100 ml
Blood urea nitrogen	28 mg/100 ml
Cholesterol	260 mg/100 ml
LDH	225 units
Uric acid	33 mg/100 ml

Study Questions

9. When can the nurse expect a therapeutic effect from an intramuscular dose of diphenylhydantoin?

10. When should the nurse administer the first dose of diphenylhydantoin by mouth?

11. Why was diphenylhydantoin ordered daily regardless of whether or not Mrs. Cooper convulsed? Should it be given if no convulsion is evident? Why?

12. What cardiovascular disorders would be contraindications to the administration of diphenylhydantoin? Why?

13. How does the serum sodium level affect seizure activity? What other serum electrolytes may also influence seizure activity?

14. What is the action of diazepam? Compare the action of diazepam with the action of diphenylhydantoin in the treatment of Mrs. Cooper's seizure disorder?

15. Which of the laboratory tests reported on the second hospital day are important in a patient with seizure activity? Why? Relate the laboratory test results to the expected need for anticonvulsants.

Third Hospital Day

Mrs. Cooper remained free from seizures during this day. She began to complain of nausea and gastric distress in the middle of the morning. Diphenylhydantoin 300 mg had been administered orally at 8:00 A.M.

Study Questions

16. Discuss the relationship between Mrs. Cooper's medications and her gastric distress.

17. What specific measures can the nurse institute to allay the gastric distress?

18. Since she is receiving an anticonvulsant orally, what aspects of Mrs. Cooper's status require careful assessment to insure consistent delivery of the drug?

Fourth Hospital Day

Mrs. Cooper had no sign of seizures but was intermittently confused.

Medical Orders

(1) Soft diet
(2) Continue intravenous fluids
(3) Dexamethasone (Decadron) 2 mg b.i.d. p.o.

Fifth and Sixth Hospital Days

The nurses observed that Mrs. Cooper was lethargic and sometimes difficult to arouse. However, she did not have any seizures. She was too sleepy to eat some of her meals and was unable to swallow her medications. Neurological checks on Mrs. Cooper were negative during this time. Several doses of her oral medications were omitted during these two days. This occurred when Mrs. Cooper put the capsule and pill in her mouth but did not swallow them because of her drowsiness. Medications were later found in the bed and on the floor.

Study Questions

19. Why was the dexamethasone dosage reduced on the fourth hospital day?

20. What medications may be responsible for Mrs. Cooper's drowsiness? Discuss other factors which may also influence this state.

21. What nursing action is indicated in relation to the lethargy and drowsiness?

22. What methods can be used to evaluate whether Mrs. Cooper can swallow?

23. If Mrs. Cooper is able to swallow, what nursing actions can be used to assist her in swallowing her pills?

24. If Mrs. Cooper is unable to swallow, what nursing actions are indicated?

25. What are the consequences of omissions in anticonvulsant drug therapy?

Seventh and Eighth Hospital Days

Occasional twitchings in the right arm were noted throughout the seventh day. At noon on the eighth day, Mrs. Cooper experienced a grand mal seizure.

Medical Orders

(1) Diazepam 5 mg IV stat. (given at 12:15 P.M.) and every 4 hours per metriset for 24 hours
(2) Continue diphenylhydantoin 100 mg t.i.d. p.o. Give diphenylhydantoin IM if patient is unable to take by mouth
(3) Increase dexamethasone to 4 mg every 8 hours

Mrs. Cooper's seizures subsided but she continued to be difficult to arouse.

Study Questions

26. What is the preferred route of administration for an anticonvulsant during a seizure when an IV route has not previously been established? Why?

27. Why is diazepam IV rather than diphenylhydantoin IV used in this situation?

28. In addition to diazepam, what other anticonvulsant drugs are often used in emergency treatment of a grand mal seizure or in status epilepticus?

29. Considering the administration of diazepam IV and Mrs. Cooper's drowsiness, what nursing judgment is necessary in regard to the administration of diphenylhydantoin?

30. Identify similarities and differences in drug therapy for the different types of convulsive disorders.

Ninth Hospital Day

Diazepam IV was discontinued and Mrs. Cooper seemed more alert and able to participate in her care. She had no difficulty taking food, fluids, and oral medications. Intravenous fluids were discontinued and, after two more days of observation without tremors or seizures, Mrs. Cooper was discharged on diphenylhydantoin 100 mg t.i.d. and dexamethasone 2 mg b.i.d.

Study Questions

31. What laboratory tests should be used to monitor Mrs. Cooper's response to long term diphenylhydantoin therapy?

32. What signs and symptoms of progressive central nervous system metastasis may be misinterpreted as side effects of diphenylhydantoin?

33. Describe the teaching needed for the administration of medications at home for a patient with seizure disorder.

34. Why is it important to include Mrs. Cooper's family when teaching about her present condition?

35. Compare the differences between a teaching plan for a patient with a seizure disorder due to metastasis of cancer and a teaching plan for a patient with "essential epilepsy".

36. How does the need for prudent mouth care relate to the long term use of diphenylhydantoin as an anticonvulsant?

37. Patients frequently discontinue medications when symptoms subside. Describe patient-teaching needed to prevent discontinuance of diphenylhydantoin by the patient or her family.

38. What side effects may prompt the patient to stop taking her diphenylhydantoin?

39. For the discharged patient, what advantage is there in the use of diphenylhydantoin instead of diazepam or phenobarbital?

40. What nonprescription drugs are known to potentiate the action of diphenylhydantoin? Name prescription drugs used in the treatment of other diseases which potentiate diphenylhydantoin action.

REFERENCES

Anticonvulsant drugs, Volume I and II. International Encyclopedic of Pharmacology and Therapeutics, Sec. 19. Pergamon Press, New York, 1973, Chapters 1 and 13.

Ausman, J. I.: New developments in anticonvulsant therapy. Postgrad. Med. 48: 122-127, 1970.

Bruya, M. A., and Bolin, R. H.: Epilepsy: a controllable disease, Part II, drug therapy and nursing care. Am. J. Nurs. 76:392-397, 1976.

Conomy, J. P., and McNamara, J. O.: Emergency management of the patient with seizures, Part II. Postgrad. Med. 55:71-74, 1974.

Cooper, C.: Anticonvulsant drugs and the epileptic's dilemma. Nursing '76, 6:44-50, 1976.

Rodman, M. J.: Drugs for treating epilepsy. R. N. 35:63-78, 1972.

Shope, J. T.: The clinical specialist in epilepsy. Nurs. Clin. N. Am. 9:761-772, 1974.

13

THE PATIENT WITH BRONCHIAL ASTHMA AND PNEUMONIA

TEXTBOOKS SUGGESTED FOR THIS STUDY

Asperheim, M. K., and Eisenhauer, L. A.: The Pharmacologic Basis of Patient Care, ed. 2. W. B. Saunders Co., Philadelphia, 1973, Chapters 9 and 16.
Bergersen, B.: Pharmacology in Nursing, ed. 13. C. V. Mosby Co., St. Louis, 1976, Chapters 16 and 20.
Brunner, L. S., and Suddarth, D.: Textbook of Medical Surgical Nursing, ed. 3. J. B. Lippincott, Philadelphia, 1975, Chapters 15 and 31.
Goodman, L., and Gilman, A. (eds.): The Pharmacological Basis of Therapeutics, ed. 5. Macmillan Co., New York, 1975, Chapters 12, 19, 29, 36, 39, 47, 49, 57, 70.
Luckmann, J., and Sorensen, K.: Medical-Surgical Nursing—A Psychophysiologic Approach. W. B. Saunders Co., Philadelphia, 1974, Chapter 71.
Rodman, M. J., and Smith, D.: Clinical Pharmacology in Nursing. J. B. Lippincott Co., Philadelphia, 1974, Chapters 19 and 41.
Shafer, K.N., et al: Medical Surgical Nursing, ed. 6. C. V. Mosby Co., St. Louis, 1975, Chapter 22.

PAST MEDICAL HISTORY

Roberta Lightfoot, a 25-year-old female, has had bronchial asthma since age seven, resulting in recurrent episodes of acute asthmatic attacks. Hospitalization was required at age 17 for severe respiratory distress, and since then increased medications including intermittent steriod therapy have been used to maintain control. Daily medications have included prednisone 5 mg: ephedrine sulfate, theophylline, and hydroxyzine hydrochloride (Marax) 1 tablet four times a day: cromolyn sodium (Aarane) four times a day: metaproterenol sulfate (Metaprel Metered Dose Inhaler) in the A.M. and at h.s. Acute episodes of asthma have occurred more frequently in the past eight years. Mrs. Lightfoot has been treated in the emergency room or hospitalized for asthma attacks once a month for the last 10 months. Mrs. Lightfoot was married at age 20, divorced a year later, and has one child, an daughter age four. Mrs. Lightfoot is presently attending college fulltime and living with her parents. The family history reveals that both parents are diabetics as well as three of her five siblings. An aunt has a 40-year history of asthma.

The present attack of asthma began when Mrs. Lightfoot awoke this morning. Symptoms of an upper respiratory infection had been present for 24 hours and wheezing on arising in the morning was not relieved by the Metaprel Metered Dose Inhaler, epinephrine (Adrenalin Chloride Solution) 0.3 ml subcutaneously, or Marax. Mrs. Lightfoot went to the emergency room of a small local hospital where treatment with methylprednisolone sodium succinate (Solu-Medrol) 8 mg and theophylline ethylenediamine (Aminophylline) 500 mg IV was ineffective in relieving her symptoms. She was hypertensive, and had tachycardia. Following consultation with her attending physician she was transferred to a large city hospital for admission to the intensive care unit.

PRESENT HOSPITAL ADMISSION

First Hospital Day

11:00 A.M. On admission to the intensive care unit Mrs. Lightfoot was orthopneic, dyspneic, lethargic, and diaphoretic. Vital signs were blood pressure 160/90, temperature 97.2^{O} F., pulse 90 and regular, and respirations 24. Her pupils were moderately dilated, eardrums normal, and nasal mucosa red and swollen. Chest examination revealed wheezes on inspiration and exhalation audible over both lung fields. Heart sounds were not audible because of the wheezes. The abdomen was markedly protuberant preventing palpation of the liver, spleen, and kidney. Examination of the extremeities revealed 1+ ankle edema on the right side and no edema on the left side. Neurological examination revealed normal deep tendon reflexes. The patient stated that she was 62 inches tall and weighed 190 pounds. The following diagnoses were made:

Acute bronchial asthma
Exogenous obesity

Medical Orders

(1) Theophylline ethylenediamine (Aminophylline) 500 mg IV every 6 hours per metriset (slow drip)
(2) Methylprednisolone (Solu-Medrol) 40 mg IV every 6 hours (give intravenous push)
(3) Diazepam (Valium) 2 mg p.o. every 4 hours p.r.n.
(4) Diazepam (Valium) 5 mg p.o. h.s. and may repeat times one
(5) Clear liquid diet
(6) Use intravenous dextrose 5% in water to keep vein open
(7) Serum sodium, potassium, chloride, complete blood count, urinalysis, arterial blood gases stat.
(8) Electrocardiogram stat.
(9) Oxygen at 2L/minute cannula or mask
(10) If patient develops severe respiratory distress, notify house physician

Study Questions

1. What is the action of theophylline ethylenediamine and why is it being administered intravenously to Mrs. Lightfoot? What is the appropriate drip rate of theophylline ethylenediamine when ordered at a "slow drip"?

2. What are the side and toxic effects of theophylline ethylenediamine and how often should the nurse evaluate Mrs. Lightfoot for their occurrence? What should be

included in this evaluation?

3. Methylprednisolone has many therapeutic actions. Which of these is most effective in treating Mrs. Lightfoot's signs and symptoms? Why?

4. How is an intravenous push injection of methylprednisolone prepared and administered by the nurse?

5. What evidence of drug toxicity is present in Mrs. Lightfoot's history?

6. What relationship is there between Mrs. Lightfoot's obesity and her history of intermittent steriod therapy?

7. What is the action of diazepam and what signs and symptoms would indicate that Mrs. Lightfoot needed this p.r.n. medication?

8. What blood gas results would lead to caution in the use of drugs such as diazepam? Why?

11:00 A.M.—3:00 P.M. Since admission Mrs. Lightfoot has had continuous inspiratory and expiratory wheezing with marked diaphoresis and an inability to assume any position but a high Fowler's. Vital signs continued to range as follows: blood pressure 158/90 - 160/90, temperature 97.2° - 97.6° F., pulse 120-148, and respirations 20-24 with wheezes audible over both lung fields.

Laboratory Results

White blood cells	19, 900 per cu mm	Serum Electrolytes	
(Differential)			
Stabs	11%	Chloride	94 mEq/L
Segs	81%	Bicarbonate	27 mEq/L
Lymphocytes	5%	Potassium	4.6 mEq/L
Monocytes	1%	Sodium	137 mEq/L
Eosinophils	2%		

Arterial blood gas studies with nasal O_2 at 2L/minute revealed pH 7.29, PaO_2 97 mm Hg, $PaCO_2$ 44 mm Hg, Base excess -6 and O_2 saturation with oxygen running 95%. Urinalysis was 2+ for sugar, negative acetone, few bacteria, and few white blood cells. Initial chest x-ray revealed an enlarged heart and minimum spotty infiltration in the lower lung fields which was compatible with peribronchial pneumonia infiltration without consolidation. Electrocardiogram showed sinus tachycardia with a heart rate of 130.

A secondary diagnosis of bilateral pneumonitis was made.

Medical Orders

(1) Furosemide (Lasix) 20 mg IV now
(2) Methylprednisolone (Solu-Medrol) 80 mg p.o. every 6 hours

(3) Cephalothin solium (Keflin) 1 gm in metriset every 4 hours after sputum specimen obtained
(4) Diphenhydramine hydrochloride, ammonium chloride, sodium citrate, chloroform and menthol (Benylin expectorant) 2 teaspoons t.i.d. p.o. p.c. and h.s.
(5) Daily weight
(6) Serum sodium, potassium, and chloride in A.M.
(7) Sputum gram stain for culture and sensitivity
(8) Fasting blood glucose in A.M.

4:45 P.M. Mrs. Lightfoot was alert and in mild respiratory distress. She coughed up small amounts of tenacious yellow sputum. Cephalothin IV was given after a sputum specimen was sent to the laboratory.

Study Questions

9. What new medications were ordered that related directly to the secondary diagnosis of pneumonia?

10. What is the action of furosemide and what instructions should the nurse administering the medication give to Mrs. Lightfoot? What are the possible reasons for its administration at this time?

11. Why was methylprednisolone increased to 80 mg every 6 hours?

12. What is the action of Benylin expectorant? Compare the actions of expectorants to antitussives and identify the value of using an expectorant at this time.

13. What is the relationship between the collection of the sputum specimen and the administration of cephalothin? How should the specimen be collected?

14. What kind of an antibiotic is cephalothin? Why was it chosen prior to the culture and sensitivity results? What are the indications for its use in the treatment of Mrs. Lightfoot?

15. Discuss the preparation and administration of cephalothin by the intravenous route.

6:30 P.M.—11:00 P.M. Mrs. Lightfoot improved considerably. She was still unable to lie down but was able to sit in bed in a semi-Fowler's position. Her cough was loose and productive of thick tenacious sputum.

11:00 P.M.-7:00 A.M. Mrs. Lightfoot slept at intervals throughout the night in a semi-Fowler's position. Her cough produced loose yellow sputum. Laboratory results showed fasting blood glucose of 151 mg %, blood pH 7.45, chloride 96 mEq/L, bicarbonate 25 mEq/L, potassium 3.8 mEq/L, and sodium 136 mEq/L. Sputum gram stain showed a moderate amount of gram-negative diplococci, gram-positive cocci, and a few gram-negative rods. Sensitivity showed pneumococci sensitive only to ampicillin and cephalexin.

Medical Orders

(1) Transfer out of intensive care unit to regular medical unit
(2) 1000 Calorie diet
(3) Repeat serum sodium, potassium, and chloride
(4) Electrocardiogram in A.M.
(5) Portable chest x-ray in A.M.
(6) Daily weight
(7) Continue same medications
(8) Potassium chloride 25 mEq (K-Lyte) twice a day p.o.
(9) Sputum culture for acid-fast bacteria times two

Study Questions

16. What side and toxic effects of cephalothin should be observed for in Mrs. Lightfoot?

17. Why was potassium chloride ordered? What is its action?

18. Discuss the factors influencing the occurrence or pneumonia in Mrs. Lightfoot. Include past medical history and medical treatment prior to admission, including the asthmatic medications that have been administered.

19. What is the purpose of the sputum specimen for acid-fast bacteria? If these results were positive, what antibiotic orders would be anticipated?

Second Hospital Day

8:00 A.M.—11:00 A.M. Mrs. Lightfoot was transferred out of the intensive care unit to a medical unit. Chest examination revealed poor aeration in both lower lung fields with no wheezing. She was coughing up copious amounts of yellowish-white mucus. Vital signs were blood pressure 120/90, pulse 128, respirations 24, and temperature 98.4^{o} F. Mrs. Lightfoot was able to stand on the scale at the bedside and her weight was 218 pounds.

Medical Orders

(1) May sit in chair
(2) Furosemide (Lasix) 40 mg p.o. stat.
(3) Increase potassium chloride 25 mEq (K-Lyte) to t.i.d. p.c.
(4) Magnesium hydroxide 7% (Milk of Magnesium) 30 ml this A.M. and p.r.n. for constipation
(5) Streptokinase-streptodornase (Varidase) 1 tablet p.c. and h.s. for 5 days
(6) Encourage water intake, not juice
(7) Measure 24-hour sputum, start this A.M.

Study Questions

20. Describe the changes in symptoms that indicate improvement in Mrs. Lightfoot's asthma. What medications have helped bring about these changes?

21. What medication may have precipitated the need for furosemide?

22. What is the relationship between the need for increased potassium chloride and the order for furosemide?

23. What is the action of strepokinase-streptodornase? How should the nurse evaluate the effectiveness of the administration of this drug?

24. What are the side effects of cephalothin and how does the nurse evaluate Mrs. Lightfoot for their occurrence?

Third and Fourth Hospital Days

Mrs. Lightfoot continued to feel better and her chest gradually began to clear. No wheezes were present but distant breath sounds were still heard in both lung fields. Vital signs remained as follows: blood pressure 128/82, pulse 88, respirations 22, and temperature 98.4° F. Sputum continued to be yellow-white and thinned out as fluid intake increased. Acid-fast sputum specimens were negative.

<u>Medical Orders</u>

(1) Discontinue cephalothin sodium (Keflin)
(2) Cephalexin monohydrate (Keflex) 500 mg t.i.d. p.c. and h.s.
(3) Discontinue IV theophylline ethylenediamine (Aminophylline)
(4) Theophylline ethylenediamine (Aminophylline) rectal suppository 500 mg h.s. every 6 hours p.r.n.
(5) Discontinue methylprednisolone (Solu-Medrol)
(6) Prednisone (Meticorten) 10 mg t.i.d. p.c. and h.s.

Study Questions

25. Why was cephalothin discontinued and cephalexin begun? What is the action of cephalexin?

26. What criteria should the nurse use to evaluate the effectiveness of cephalexin?

27. Why was theophylline ethylenediamine IV changed to a suppository? How should the nurse determine when to give this medication to Mrs. Lightfoot?

28. Discuss the change of order from methylprednisolone to prednisone. What is the action of each of these medications and what has occurred to indicate the change from intravenous to oral medication?

29. What relationship, if any, is there between the administration of the steroid and the occurrence of pneumonia?

30. What evidence is present of the effectiveness of medication therapy in the treatment of pneumonia? What difference is there between this type of response and the response of patients with pneumonia prior to the use of antibiotic therapy?

31. What precautions are advised in the use of antibiotic therapy to promote effective destruction of pathogens? Discuss the need for continued research of new antibiotics and relate it to the reason why penicillin was not used to treat Mrs. Lightfoot's pneumonia.

Fifth Hospital Day

Mrs. Lightfoot's chest x-ray picture taken the previous day showed minimal peribronchial pneumonia infiltrate with no evidence of consolidation of pleural effusion. Comparison to the previous x-ray study showed general clearing of the pneumonic process. She continued to respond well to antibiotic therapy and was expectorating large amounts of tenacious whitish-yellow sputum. Chest examination revealed fine rales in both lower lung bases. Vital signs ranged as follows: blood pressure 124/72 - 130/80, pulse 68-92, respirations 22-24, temperature 98.2° - 99.2° F. Repeated white blood count showed the following:

White blood count	18,800 per cu mm
(Differential)	
Stabs	3%
Segs	86%
Lymphocytes	8%
Monocytes	3%
Eosinophils	0%

An electrocardiogram showed a normal tracing. Mrs. Lightfoot's weight on the fifth hospital day was 217 pounds and she indicated that she gained weight very easily when taking prednisone. She was up and about with no dyspnea or wheezing. Discharge was scheduled for the following day.

Discharge Orders

(1) 1000 calorie low-salt diet
(2) Cephalexin monohydrate (Keflex) 500 mg t.i.d. p.c. and h.s.#20
(3) Ephedrine sulfate, theophylline, and hydroxyzine hydrochloride (Marax) 1 tablet t.i.d. p.c. and h.s.#60
(4) Prednisone (Meticorten) 10 mg t.i.d. p.c. and h.s.#30
(5) Diphenhydramine hydrochloride, ammonium chloride, sodium citrate, chloroform, and menthol (Benylin expectorant) 2 teaspoons t.i.d. p.c. and h.s. 4 oz.
(6) Potassium chloride 25 mEq (K-Lyte) b.i.d. p.c. 2 weeks supply
(7) Diazepam (Valium) 5 mg h.s.# 30
(8) Theophylline ethylenediamine (Aminophylline) rectal suppository 500 mg 1 h.s. daily
(9) Streptokinase-streptodornase (Varidase) 1 tablet t.i.d. p.c. and h.s.# 20
(10) Instruct patient in deep breathing and pursed lip breathing exercises

Study Questions

32. What evidence is there of further progress in the clearing of the pneumonia?

33. Compare the white blood count and differential to that done on admission. The action of what medication is specifically related to these changes?

34. What is the relationship between weight gain and the administration of prednisone? What instructions can be given Mrs. Lightfoot to assist her in decreasing this effect?

35. Separate the discharge medications ordered for Mrs. Lightfoot into two groups—those aimed at further treatment of pneumonia and those included in the asthmatic therapy. What is the action of each medication?

36. How should Mrs. Lightfoot be instructed in the use of these medications? Consider methods that can be used to insure that Mrs. Lightfoot takes the right medications at the correct times each day.

37. What instructions should be included about taking the entire amount of cephalexin ordered? Why is this aspect important?

38. The nondiscriminating action of many antibiotics results in destruction of nonpathogenic body organisms as well as pathogens. What problems can occur because of these actions?

39. Discuss the positive and negative effects of IPPB and inhalation medications in the treatment of bronchial asthma and pneumonia.

REFERENCES

Deliee, Sr., S., and Cardoni, A. A.: Antimicrobials: team effort keeps wonder drugs wonderful, N '75, 5:22-27, 1975.

Dewey, J.: 18 ways to live with asthma, N '75, 5:48-51, 1975.

Geolot, D. H., and McKenney, N.P.: Administering parenteral drugs, Am. J. Nurs. 75:788-793, 1975.

Leary, J. A., Vassela, D. M., and Yeaw, E.M.: Self-administered medication, Am. J. Nurs., 71:1193-1194, 1971.

Lee, R.V.: Antimicrobial therapy, Am. J. Nurs., 73:2044-2048, 1973.

Rodman, M. J.: Drugs for bacterial pneumonias, R.N. 34:55-62, 1971.

Tobey, L., and Covinton, T.: Antimicrobial drug interactions, Am. J. Nurs., 75:1470-1473, 1975.

14

THE PATIENT WITH SEPTICEMIA

TEXTBOOKS SUGGESTED FOR THIS STUDY

Asperheim, M. K., and Eisenhauer, L. A.: The Pharmacologic Basis of Patient Care, ed. 2. W. B. Saunders Co., Philadelphia, 1973, Chapters 6, 9, 11, 12, and 15.

Bergersen, B.: Pharmacology in Nursing, ed. 13. C. V. Mosby Co., St. Louis, 1976, Chapters 9, 11, 18, 20, and 29.

Brunner, L. S., and Suddarth, D.: Textbook of Medical Surgical Nursing, ed. 3. J. B. Lippincott Co., Philadelphia, 1975, Chapters 10 and 37.

Goodman, L., and Gilman, A. (eds.): The Pharmacological Basis of Therapeutics, ed. 5. Macmillan Co., New York, 1975, Chapters 15, 24, 36, 57, 58, 70, 73, and 74.

Luckmann, J., and Sorensen, K.: Medical-Surgical Nursing — A Psychophysiologic Approach. W. B. Saunders Co., Philadelphia, 1974, Chapter 26.

Rodman, M. J., and Smith, D.: Pharmacology and Drug Therapy in Nursing. J. B. Lippincott Co., Philadelphia, 1974, Chapters 13, 17, 23, 41, and 49.

Shafer, K. N., et al.: Medical Surgical Nursing, ed. 6. C. V. Mosby Co., St. Louis, 1975, Chapter 19.

PRESENT HOSPITAL ADMISSION

Mr. Williams, a 30-year-old man, was brought to the emergency room at 2:00 A.M. by his family. He had sustained multiple stab wounds in a fight. The wounds were in the upper abdomen, back, and both thighs. On admission, hemoglobin was 14.6 gm/100 ml, hematocrit 45%, and white blood count 3800 per cu mm. Vital signs were temperature 102.4° F., pulse 96, respirations 36, and blood pressure 80/60. X-ray studies showed a small amount of fluid within the upper abdomen which suggested bleeding into the abdominal cavity from the stab wound in the abdomen. Mr. Williams was very restless and was complaining of pain in his abdomen and back. He vomited a large amount of white liquid. His family said he had been healthy most of his life except for five years ago when he had "stomach trouble" and took milk and antacids. He smoked an average of one pack of cigarettes a day and drank alcoholic beverages, usually on the weekend. He was employed as a janitor in a local factory. He was single and lived with his parents and younger siblings.

First Hospital Day

Mr. Williams was taken to surgery for suturing of the stab wounds. Because of the nature of the wounds, it was necessary for the physician to perform an exploratory laparotomy. During the laparotomy a perforation of the splenic flexure of the colon was found, and a colostomy was done. There was evidence of peritonitis throughout the entire abdomen.

6:00 A.M. Mr. Williams was admitted to the Intensive Care Unit. His vital signs were pulse 140, respirations 44, and blood pressure 86/70. He was receiving a unit of whole blood and 5% glucose in water 1000 ml IV. He had a nasogastric tube and an indwelling catheter in the urinary bladder and a central venous pressure line in place with a reading of 3.0 cm. He appeared to be in a state of semiconsciousness.

Medical Orders

(1) Meperidine hydrochloride (Demerol) 100 mg IM every 4 hours p.r.n. for pain
(2) Ampicillin (Polycillin) 1.0 gm (IV metriset) every 6 hours
(3) Gentamycin sulfate (Garamycin) 80 mg (IV metriset) every 6 hours
(4) Intravenous fluids as follows for 24 hours:
 3000 ml of 5% glucose in water
 1000 ml of 5% glucose in normal saline with 40 mEq potassium chloride
(5) Hydrocortisone sodium succinate (Solu-Cortef) 300 mg added to each 1000 ml of intravenous fluids
(6) Oxygen at 6 L per minute
(7) Intake and output
(8) Monitor urinary output every hour
(9) Vital signs every 15 minutes
(10) Central venous pressure every 15 minutes
(11) Hemoglobin, hematocrit, serum electrolytes, carbon dioxide, and BUN every day

Study Questions

1. Why have two different antibiotics been ordered for Mr. Williams? Describe the action of each.

2. Explain the difference between bactericidal and bacteriostatic actions of antibiotics.

3. What is meant by a broad-spectrum antibiotic?

4. How does the dose of ampicillin that was ordered for Mr. Williams compare with the usual dose?

5. How would the nurse prepare and administer the antibiotics by metriset?

6. Explain why it was necessary to order the large quantity of intravenous fluids?

7. What is the purpose of adding potassium chloride to one IV bottle?

8. Discuss why a cortisone preparation was indicated for Mr. Williams.

9. What criteria would the nurse use to evaluate the effectiveness of steroid administration in the treatment of Mr. Williams?

10. Compare the relative danger of side effects from the glucocorticoids administered in an emergency situation to those administered over a long period of time.

7:00 A.M. Mr. Williams was perspiring profusely, his skin was cold, and his color was ashen. His temperature was 103° F. (rectally), pulse 150, respirations 60, central venous pressure 0, and urinary output 0. The nurse could not hear the blood pressure. The physician was notified and, after examining the patient, made the diagnosis of septic shock.

Medical Orders

500 ml 5% glucose in normal saline intravenous with levarterenol bitartrate (Levophed Bitartrate) 4 mg. Regulate drops to maintain systolic blood pressure at 90 or above.

Study Questions

11. Describe the action of levarterenol.

12. Levarterenol is called a vasopressor drug. What does this mean?

13. What is the danger of giving vasopressors without sufficient fluid replacement?

14. Describe how the nurse would monitor levarterenol administration in relation to blood pressure.

15. How soon could the nurse expect a change in the blood pressure with the administration of levarterenol?

16. How would the nurse evaluate the effectiveness of levarterenol?

17. Why are vasopressor drugs used only in emergency situations?

12:00 P.M. Mrs. Williams' skin was warm. His temperature was 103° F. (rectally), pulse 144, respirations 52, systolic blood pressure 90, central venous pressure 4.0 cm, and the last hourly urinary output 25 ml. The nurse noted a small amount of bright bloody drainage when she reinforced the abdominal dressing. The patient began to ask the nurse about the reason for all his treatments and complained once of mild abdominal pain.

Study Questions

18. Describe the action of meperidine hydrochloride. Should it be administered at this time?

19. What problems may occur if levarterenol infiltrates into the tissues surrounding the vein?

8:00 P.M. Mr. Williams' temperature remained elevated as did his pulse and respirations. There was no further bleeding noted from the abdominal incision. The nasogastric tube drained a small amount of greenish liquid and the abdomen was soft. Mr. Williams continued to be restless and tried to get out of bed. The nurse changed his position frequently, but he could not cooperate enough to cough and deep breathe. At intervals the nurse spoke with the family who waited anxiously.

Second Hospital Day

6:00 A.M. 24-Hour Intake and Output

Intake:	4800 ml IV	Output:	500 ml Urine
			300 ml Gastric Drainage

Laboratory Results (8:00 A.M.)

Hemoglobin	13.4 gm/100 ml
Hematocrit	43%
Blood urea nitrogen	32 mg/100 ml
Sodium	139 mEq/L
Potassium	4.9 mEq/L
Chloride	100 mEq/L
Carbon dioxide	17 mEq/L

10:00 A.M. The nurse was unable to hear the blood pressure. Mr. Williams' temperature was 104.4° F. (rectally), pulse 140, respirations 40, central venous pressure 2.0 cm, and his skin was cold and clammy.

Medical Orders

(1) Continue levarterenol bitartrate (Levophed Bitartrate) to maintain a systolic blood pressure of 90 or above
(2) Blood culture stat.
(3) Repeat hemoglobin, hematocrit, serum electrolytes, carbon dioxide, and BUN

Third Hospital Day

24-Hour Intake and Output

Intake:	5000 ml IV	Output:	2025 ml Urine
			500 ml Gastric Drainage

8:00 A.M. During the previous afternoon, Mr. Williams' blood pressure became audible and stabilized around 100/40. His temperature was 102° F. (rectally), pulse 120, respirations 30, and central venous pressure 4.5 cm. He was less restless and somewhat confused but he could cooperate in turning.

Laboratory Results

Hemoglobin	13 gm/100 ml
Hematocrit	42%
Blood urea nitrogen	25 mg/100 ml

Sodium	133 mEq/L
Potassium	4.5 mEq/L
Chloride	90 mEq/L
Carbon dioxide	25 mEq/L
Blood culture	Escherichia coli

Medical Orders

(1) Decrease hydrocortisone sodium succinate (Solu-Cortef) to 100 mg in each 1000 ml of IV fluids
(2) Decrease oxygen to 4 L per minute
(3) Irrigate incision with warm saline b.i.d.
(4) Change dressing b.i.d.

Study Questions

20. Why was the hydrocortisone sodium succinate decreased?

21. What symptoms would the nurse look for if the hydrocortisone sodium succinate was withdrawn suddenly rather than gradually?

22. Discuss the signs of effectiveness of the treatment of the septic shock.

Fifth Hospital Day

24-Hour Intake and Output

Intake:	Output:
4000 ml IV	2675 ml Urine
	1320 ml Gastric Drainage

8:00 A.M. As the nurse changed the dressing she noted that the incision was not healing well. The suture line was inflamed and there was purulent drainage present which appeared to contain fecal material. Vital signs were temperature 100° F. (rectally), pulse 112, respirations 24, and blood pressure 110/90. Mr. Williams was now oriented to time and place.

Medical Orders

Culture and sensitivity of drainage from incision

Study Questions

23. In addition to the administration of antibiotics, what other nursing care should be carried out to prevent further pathogenic microorganism growth in Mr. Williams' incision?

24. How can the nurse protect herself and other patients from the spread of the pathogens?

Seventh Hospital Day

8:00 A.M. Mr. Williams continued to improve. His vital signs stabilized and his gastric drainage began to decrease. His wound was less inflamed, and there was less purulent drainage present.

Laboratory Results

Culture of drainage from incision revealed Escherichia coli
Sensitive to: ampicillin, chloramphenicol, erythromycin, gentamycin, kenamycin, streptomycin, and tetracycline
Resistant to: demeclocycline, lincomycin, and penicillin

Medical Orders

(1) Decrease ampicillin (Polycillin) to 500 mg IV every 6 hours
(2) Decrease gentamycin sulfate (Garamycin) to 40 mg IV every 6 hours

12:00 P.M. Mr. Williams began to perspire profusely and became very restless and apprehensive. He called the nurse who immediately checked his vital signs. His temperature was 104.4° F. (rectally), pulse 120, respirations 40, central venous pressure 1.5 cm, and blood pressure inaudible. The nurse restarted the levarterenol and notified the physician of the change in Mr. Williams' condition. She also notified the family of the change. In the meantime she tried to comfort and reassure Mr. Williams.

Medical Orders

(1) Whole blood 500 ml stat.
(2) Increase hydrocortisone sodium succinate (Solu-Cortef) to 200 mg in each 1000 ml of intravenous fluids
(3) Increase ampicillin (Polycillin) to 1.0 gm IV every 6 hours
(4) Increase gentamycin sulfate (Garamycin) to 80 mg IV every 6 hours
(5) Blood culture stat.

Study Questions

25. What changes in Mr. Williams' condition made it necessary to increase the antibiotics?

26. What criteria did the nurse use that indicated she needed to restart the levarterenol?

27. Explain the use of culture and sensitivity studies when antibiotics are used for treatment.

8:00 P.M. Mr. Williams' pulse was 110, respirations 32, blood pressure 100/62, and central venous pressure 3.0 cm. He was less restless and was able to speak with his family.

Ninth Hospital Day

8:00 A.M. Mr. Williams was more cooperative. He was able to cough up some mucus. The wound continued to have a small amount of purulent drainage. Mr. Williams complained of pain at intervals, and the nurse administered meperidine hydrochloride. The gentamycin and hydrocortisone sodium succinate were again decreased, and the oxygen was discontinued. The blood culture continued to show Escherichia coli.

Tenth Hospital Day

8:00 A.M. The nasogastric tube was removed and Mr. Williams was given liquids by mouth. He tolerated the liquids well and did not complain of nausea or distention. His temperature was 101° F. (rectally), pulse 100, respirations 24, blood pressure 120/80, and central venous pressure 4.5 cm.

Medical Orders

(1) Discontinue central venous pressure line
(2) Omit levarterenol bitartrate (Levophed Bitartrate)
(3) Give intravenous fluids as follows for 24 hours:
    (a) 1000 ml of 5% glucose in normal saline with 40 mEq potassium chloride
    (b) 1000 ml of 5% glucose in water with 1 ampule vitamins B and C (Berocca-C)
    (c) 1000 ml of 5% glucose in normal saline
(4) Decrease hydrocortisone sodium succinate (Solu-Cortef) to 50 mg added to each 1000 ml of IV fluids
(5) Omit meperidine hydrochloride (Demerol)
(6) Pentazocine hydrochloride (Talwin) 30 mg IM every 4 hours p.r.n. for pain

Study Questions

28. What observations of Mr. Williams should the nurse make following the discontinuation of levarterenol bitartrate?

29. Why was it necessary to give vitamins B and C?

30. Compare the analgesic properties of pentazocine hydrochloride with those of meperidine hydrochloride.

31. What measures can the nurse use to enhance the use of an analgesic?

32. Discuss drug dependence that may develop with the use of pentazocine.

Fourteenth Hospital Day

8:00 A.M. Mr. Williams continued to take fluids by mouth, and his intake and output were adequate. His temperature was 100° F. (orally), pulse 110, respirations 22, and blood pressure 120/80.

Laboratory and X-ray Results

Hemoglobin	9.9 gm/100 ml
Hematocrit	29%
White blood count	12,770 per cu mm
Sodium	138 mEq/L
Potassium	3.5 mEq/L
Chloride	93 mEq/L
Blood urea nitrogen	13 mg/100 ml
Carbon dioxide	22 mEq/L
Chest and abdomen	clear

Medical Orders

Whole blood 500 ml today and tomorrow

Study Question

33. What indications are there for the administration of blood?

Sixteenth Hospital Day

10:00 A.M. Mr. Williams was transferred from the Intensive Care Unit to a surgical floor. He was apprehensive about leaving the ICU, so a nurse from the surgical floor came to the ICU to orient him to the new floor prior to the transfer. After he was transferred, he was given a soft diet. The nurse attached a bag to the colostomy, which was functioning well. Intravenous fluids were decreased to 1000 ml daily. Mr. Williams' vital signs were temperature 100° F. (orally), pulse 100, respirations 20, and blood pressure 110/70.

Medical Orders

(1) Discontinue hydrocortisone sodium succinate (Solu-Cortef) and gentamycin sulfate (Garamycin)
(2) Ampicillin (Polycillin) 500 mg IM every 6 hours

Study Questions

34. Compare the advantages and disadvantages of administering antibiotics intravenously with those of administering them intramuscularly.

35. What measures could the nurse use to decrease discomfort with intramuscular injections?

Twentieth Hospital Day

8:00 A.M. Mr. Williams was much stronger and was able to get out of bed. His incision was healing well. He was alert and responsive. His vital signs were temperature 99° F., pulse 90, respirations 20, and blood pressure 110/80. The indwelling catheter and the intravenous fluids were discontinued. Mr. Williams seldom required medication for pain, and he tolerated his regular diet well. He and the nurse worked together as he learned to care for his colostomy. He said he was "tired of getting shots" and wanted "pills" instead.

Laboratory Results

Hemoglobin	12 gm/100 ml
Hematocrit	38%
White blood count	9,700 per cu mm

Study Question

36. Explain patient-teaching the nurse could do as to the advantage of giving antibiotics intramuscularly rather than orally.

Twenty-fourth Hospital Day

8:00 A.M. Mr. Williams' vital signs were temperature 98.6° F., pulse 80, respirations 20, and blood pressure 110/80. The ampicillin was discontinued. The nurse prepared the patient for discharge.

12:00 P.M. Mr. Williams was discharged accompanied by his family. He was to return in one month for follow-up care. Surgery to close the colostomy was to be scheduled for a later date.

REFERENCES

A guide to admixture compatibility, Part I, R.N. 36:32-37, 1973; Part II, R.N. 36: 36-40, 1973; Part III, R.N. 36:32-37.

Cluff, L. E., and Deal, W. B.: Bacteriuria and bacteremia. Hosp. Manage. 10:62-79, 1974.

Frank, J. T.: Septic shock. Drug Intel. Clin. Pharm. 7:25-32, 1973.

Giolot, D. H., and McKinney, N. P.: Administering parenteral drugs. Am. J. Nurs. 75:788-793, 1975.

Lewis, J. G.: Gram-negative bacteraemia. Nurs. Mirror, 139:47-49, 1974.

Moyer, J. H., and Mills, L. C.: Vasopressor agents in shock. Am. J. Nurs. 75:620-625, 1975.

Rodman, M. J.: Antimicrobial drugs for septicemia. R. N. 39:67-68, 1976.

Rodman, M. J.: Fighting the second most frequent infections. Part II, R. N. 38:91-92 and 95, 1975.

Septicemia in a changing world. Emerg. Med. 5:70-93, 1973.

15

THE PATIENT WITH A MYOCARDIAL INFARCTION

TEXTBOOKS SUGGESTED FOR THIS STUDY

Asperheim, K., and Eisenhauer, A.: The Pharmacologic Basis of Patient Care. W. B. Saunders Co., Philadelphia, 1973. Chapters 3 and 19.

Bergerson, B.: Pharmacology in Nursing, ed. 13. C. V. Mosby Co., St. Louis, 1976, Chapters 10, 11, and 12.

Brunner, L. S., and Suddarth, D. S.: Textbook of Medical-Surgical Nursing. J. B. Lippincott Co., 1975, Chapters 17, 18, and 19.

Goodman, L., and Gilman, A., (eds.): The Pharmacological Basis of Therapeutics, ed. 5. Macmillan Co., New York, 1975, Chapters 12, 15, 32, 34, and 49.

Johns, M. P.: Pharmacodynamics and Patient Care. C. V. Mosby Co., St. Louis, 1974, Chapter 10.

Luckmann, J., and Sorensen, K.: Medical-Surgical Nursing—A Psychophysiologic Approach. W. B. Saunders Co., Philadelphia, 1974, Chapters 49, 50, and 51.

Rodman, M. J.: Clinical Pharmacology in Nurisng. J. B. Lippincott Co., Philadelphia, 1974, Chapters 29 and 30.

Shafer, K., et al: Medical-Surgical Nursing, ed. 6. C. V. Mosby Co., St. Louis, 1975, Chapter 17.

PAST MEDICAL HISTORY

Carl Roberts, a 56-year-old man, became dizzy while working as a television repairman at the Salvation Army and collapsed to the ground. He complained of crushing substernal chest pain while being placed in an ambulance and was very diaphoretic and short of breath when he arrived at the medical center. Mr. Roberts had no previous history of cardiac disease and no symptoms of heart problems. He smoked one-and-a-half packs of cigarettes per day and had a history of heavy alcohol ingestion.

PRESENT HOSPITAL ADMISSION

First Hospital Day

Mr. Roberts was admitted to the coronary care unit following an emergency electrocardiogram which showed changes consistent with a probable acute anteroseptal lateral myocardial infarction. Morphine administered intravenously in the emergency room was effective in controlling his chest pain and dyspnea. Mr. Roberts was responsive and his skin was warm and dry on entering the coronary care unit. Vital signs were blood pressure 116/84, pulse 84, and respirations 22.

Medical Orders

(1) Intravenous 5% dextrose in water at 5-10 drops per minute
(2) Soft 1000 mg sodium diet
(3) Bedrest on cardiac monitor
(4) ECG on the next two days
(5) Lidocaine (Xylocaine) 50 mg IV bolus p.r.n. for significant premature ventricular contractions (PVC'S); if unrelieved, give lidocaine 2-4 mg per minute in an intravenous drip
(6) Atropine 0.5 mg IV p.r.n. for pulse rate below 45 beats per minute
(7) Procainamide hydrochloride (Pronestyl) 2-4 mg per minute IV for PVC's resistant to lidocaine
(8) Nitroglycerin (Nitrostat) 0.4 mg sublingual p.r.n. for anginal chest pain
(9) Morphine sulphate 5-10 mg IV every 3 hours p.r.n. for severe chest pain
(10) Acetaminophen (Tylenol) 650 mg p.o. every 4 hours p.r.n. for moderate pain
(11) Dioctyl sodium sulfosuccinate (Colace) 100 mg p.o. b.i.d.
(12) Diazepam (Valium) 5 mg p.o. every 4 hours p.r.n. for apprehension
(13) Oxygen 2-4 L per minute by nasal prongs p.r.n.
(14) SGOT, CPK, stat. and tomorrow morning
(15) Serum potassium, serum sodium, and serum chloride stat.

Study Questions

1. The use of medications in the coronary care unit is different from the use of medications on regular hospital units. Compare the nurses' role and the hospital policies regarding medication administration in each of these areas.

2. Why was a slow intravenous infusion ordered for Mr. Roberts?

3. Describe the pharmacological actions of lidocaine and discuss its use in Mr. Roberts' therapy.

4. Describe what is meant by the term "bolus."

5. Lidocaine has been ordered for the treatment of significant premature ventricular contractions (PVC's). What criteria should be used to determine which PVC's should be treated with intravenous lidocaine?

6. Relate the length of action of lidocaine to the use of both intermittent and continuous intravenous infusions of this medication.

7. Discuss the similarities and differences in the use of atropine as a preoperative medication and as an antiarrhythmic agent.

8. When atropine is used to treat a bradycardia, what side effects should the nurse tell the patient to expect?

9. How does the pharmacological action of procainamide differ from that of lidocaine?

10. How does nitroglycerin act to relieve anginal chest pain?

11. Why is morphine one of the most frequently prescribed narcotics for the relief of pain associated with myocardial infarction?

12. Why may intramuscular injections be contraindicated for patients who have the diagnosis of myocardial infarction?

13. What is the action of acetaminophen? Why was it ordered for pain for Mr. Roberts in addition to the nitroglycerin and morphine? Why is it preferable to other similar analgesics?

14. Discuss the pharmacological action of dioctyl sodium sulfosuccinate and the reason it was ordered b.i.d. for Mr. Roberts.

2:00 P.M. Mr. Robert's monitor pattern began to show frequent PVC's with occasional coupling. An IV bolus of lidocaine 50 mg was administered.

2:10 P.M. The PVC's persisted and an intravenous infusion of lidocaine 3 mg per minute was started.

2:20 P.M. Mr. Roberts continued to have frequent PVC's with no response to lidocaine. The lidocaine infusion was stopeed and an IV infusion of procainamide 3 mg per minute was started.

2:30 P.M. Mr. Robert's vital signs remained stable: blood pressure 112/70, pulse 80, and respirations 20, and he was alert and responsive. He continued to have the same ventricular irritability. The nurse reduced the procainamide infusion to 2 mg per minute and added an infusion of lidocaine 2 mg per minute. This combination reduced Mr. Robert's cardiac irritability, and only rare PVC's were noted.

3:00 P.M. The lidocaine and procainamide infusions were discontinued and a slow drip of dextrose 5% in water was connected to the intravenous site.

Study Questions

15. Describe the effectiveness of lidocaine in the treatment of Mr. Robert's PVC's.

16. What decisions were made by the nurse in carrying out the medical orders for the treatment of Mr. Roberts' ventricular irritability?

17. Compare the combined pharmacological effect of lidocaine and procainamide when given together to the effects of each drug given separately.

18. How does the nurse evaluate the need for antiarrhythmic medications for Mr. Roberts?

19. Describe the possible methods of administering Mr. Roberts' intravenous lidocaine and procainamide considering the fact that he only had one intravenous infusion rate.

4:00 P.M. Although Mr. Roberts' ventricular arrhythmias had subsided, he complained of substernal chest pain. He was given nitroglycerin 0.4 mg sublingually. His chest pain persisted and at 4:15 P.M. morphine 5 mg was given which provided adequate relief.

5:00 P.M. Mr. Roberts' vital signs remained stable: blood pressure 124/90, pulse 76, and respirations 18, and he was resting comfortably. He appeared apprehensive about his condition and diazepam 5 mg was given orally. Occasional PVC's began to occur with some coupling and the nurse started an intravenous infusion of procainamide 2 mg per minute and lidocaine 1 mg per minute.

6:00 P.M.—12:00 P.M. Mr. Roberts appeared less apprehensive and was able to take short naps during the early evening. The intravenous administration of lidocaine and procainamide reduced his ventricular irritability; however, he began to have PVC's whenever the medications were discontinued for more than 30 minutes. At 8:00 P.M. he began to have another episode of chest pain which was relieved by an intravenous injection of morphine 5 mg. He was able to rest comfortably when the pain subsided but was noted to become dyspneic and cyanotic with only a small amount of exertion. Oxygen was started at 2 L per minute by nasal prongs and by 10:00 P.M. Mr. Roberts was sleeping restfully.

Study Questions

20. Why was nitroglycerin given when Mr. Roberts first complained of pain? Was this an appropriate nursing action or should he have been given morphine first? Why?

21. The effective alleviation of myocardial infarction pain by medications prevents what complicating physiological reactions?

22. What are the advantages of administering Mr. Roberts' morphine intravenously? What precautions must the nurse take during administration?

23. How does the nurse determine which dosage of morphine should be administered? Discuss the legality of these methods of ordering analgesics.

24. Discuss the therapeutic effects of diazepam and describe its use in Mr. Roberts' treatment.

25. What is the value of administering oxygen to a patient who has had a myocardial infarction? What were the indications for its use in the treatment of Mr. Roberts?

Second Hospital Day

12:00 P.M.—7:30 A.M. During the night Mr. Roberts had two episodes of substernal chest pain which were relieved by morphine. His ventricular irritability decreased and he did not receive antiarrhythmic drugs after 2:00 A.M. He slept comfortably with his oxygen running continuously at 2 liters per minute.

Laboratory Results (7:30 A.M.)

Serum potassium	6.0 mEq/L
Serum sodium	133 mEq/L
Serum chloride	96 mEq/L
SGOT	38 units
LDH	174 units
CPK	302 units

7:30 A.M. Mr. Roberts' vital signs remained stable: temperature 97.2^{o}F., blood pressure 120/90, pulse 84, and respirations 22. He complained of a dull aching pain in his chest which was relieved by acetaminophen 650 mg given orally. He appeared to be apprehensive and refused to have any morning care.

10:00 A.M. Mr. Roberts' apprehension increased and he becamse diaphoretic, appeared short of breath, and vomited. He complained of pain in his chest and his monitor pattern showed frequent PVC's. His blood pressure was 98/60, pulse 88, and respirations 28. Morphine 5 mg was administered IV, his oxygen was increased to 4 L per minute, and lidocaine 2 mg per minute and procainamide 2 mg per minute were started intravenously. His physician was notified and a stat. ECG was done.

10:30 A.M. Mr. Roberts responded well to treatment and rested comfortably with no further complaints of pain. He was no longer diaphoretic and his respirations were slow and rhythmic at 18 per minute. The ECG report showed an evolving myocardial infarction with a new interventricular conduction defect resembling left bundle branch block.

Study Questions

26. During Mr. Roberts' 10:00 A.M. episode of chest pain, dyspnea, and diaphoresis, the nurse made several observations and responded by administering specific medications. Describe those observations and indicate the reasons each medication was given.

27. List the order of priority for carrying out the nursing actions which were performed at 10:00 A.M.

28. Mr. Roberts was described as being apprehensive at 10:00 A.M. Although several medications were administered, diazepam which was ordered for apprehension was not given. Was it an appropriate nursing action to omit diazepam at this time? Why?

12:00 P.M.—8:00 P.M. Mr. Roberts had two more episodes of chest pain which were relieved by intravenous morphine. One episode of frequent PVC's was terminated by an intravenous bolus of lidocaine 50 mg. Mr. Roberts' appetite was poor and he tolerated only frequent sips of fruit juice.

Third Hospital Day

4:00 A.M. A dull aching chest pain awakened Mr. Roberts. Although he stated that he was not short of breath, he appeared tachypneic with respirations at 32 per minute. His blood pressure was 120/90 and pulse 82. He was given acetaminophen 650 mg p.o. which relieved his pain. His oxygen which had been reduced to 2 L per minute was increased to 4 L per minute.

7:00 A.M. Mr. Roberts slept following his episode of chest pain and awakened feeling well rested. A few bibasilar rales were noticed for the first time. His skin was warm and dry and his color was described as good.

Laboratory Results

SGOT	341 units
LDH	936 units
CPK	3340 units

3:00 P.M.—10:00 P.M. Mr. Roberts' condition remained stable during the day. He did not require any medication for pain. At 4:45 P.M. he was given lidocaine 50 mg intravenously for a short run of ventricular tachycardia. He rested comfortably in bed and ate most of his dinner stating, "my appetite is slowly coming back." His oxygen was discontinued at 6:00 P.M., his skin remained warm and dry, and his color was good.

Study Questions

29. What criteria were used by Mr. Roberts' nurse in determining what analgesic to administer for the 4:00 A.M. episode of chest pain?

30. Compare the absorption rate and length of action between an oral pain medication and pain medication given intravenously.

31. Discuss the potential need for additional arrhythmia medications in light of Mr. Roberts' 8:00 A.M. serum enzyme levels.

32. Mr. Roberts received a bolus of lidocaine for a very short run of ventricular tachycardia. Would an acceptable alternative for his nurse have been to hold his medication until she was able to determine if this was just an isolated irregularity? Why?

Fourth Hospital Day

7:00 A.M.—1:00 P.M. Mr. Roberts slept comfortably during the night. His vital signs remained stable, he ate breakfast, and appeared cheerful during his bath. At 11:00 A.M. his nurse noticed that he was very quiet and was anxiously watching his monitor. During conversation, Mr. Roberts told her that he overheard his doctor saying that he was going to be transferred out of the coronary care unit. He said, "They won't watch my heart like you nurses do. I don't want to go." After spending several minutes describing the unit to which he would be transferred and the telemetry monitoring system, his nurse gave him diazepam 5 mg orally. By noontime he appeared relaxed and following lunch he was resting comfortably reading the newspaper.

3:00 P.M. Mr. Roberts was transferred to the intermediate care unit. His vital signs were stable: blood pressure 100/84, pulse 84, and respirations 20. His skin was warm and dry and he had a few bibasilar rales. He had no complaints of chest pain or dyspnea and accepted the transfer with no further expressions of anxiety.

11:00 P.M. An aching chest pain which radiated to his left arm awakened Mr. Roberts and he notified his nurse. She gave him nitroglycerin 0.4 mg sublingually, following which the pain subsided and he rested comfortably the rest of the evening.

Study Questions

33. What nursing observations and actions occurred at 11:00 A.M.? Discuss the use of diazepam at that time including its effectiveness.

34. How did Mr. Roberts' episode of pain at 11:00 P.M. differ from his previous episodes of chest pain? Describe the pharmacological actions of nitroglycerin that resulted in the relief of that pain.

Progress Report

During the next two weeks, Mr. Roberts' condition steadily improved. He had no more episodes of cardiac irritability and his activity was gradually increased following a planned program for coronary rehabilitation. He did have occasional chest pain which was readily relieved by nitroglycerin. He was discharged on the 21st hospital day.

<u>Discharge Orders</u>

(1) Nitroglycerin (Nitrostat) 0.4 mg sublingual p.r.n. for anginal pain
(2) No-added-salt 3000 Calorie diet
(3) Return to medical clinic in one week

Study Questions

35. Nitroglycerin was ordered p.r.n. for Mr. Roberts. How should the use of a p.r.n. medication be explained to him?

36. What instructions should be included while teaching the sublingual administration of nitroglycerin?

37. What should Mr. Roberts be told about the effects of nitroglycerin?

38. Since the potency of nitroglycerin is affected by time, heat, light, air, and moisture, what instructions related to these factors should be included in Mr. Roberts' teaching plan?

REFERENCES

Allendorf, E. E., and Keegan, M. H.: Teaching patients about nitroglycerin, Am. J. Nurs., 75:1168-1170, 1975.

Biddle, T. L., and Yu, P. N.: Understanding and treating arrhythmias accompanying myocardial infarctions. Nurs. Clin. N. A., 7:481-490, 1972.

Deberry, P., Jefferies, L., and Light, M.: Teaching cardiac patients to manage medications. Am. J. Nurs., 75:2191-2193, 1975.

DiPalma, J. T.: Oxygen as drug therapy. R.N. 34:49-51, 1971.

Kise, M. S.: Drug therapy in the treatment of angina pectoris. Nurs. Clin. N. A., 11:309-318, 1976.

Kratz, A. M., and Kratz, J. L.: Cardiac drugs today—vasodilators. Nursing '73, 3:33-37, 1973.

Levitt, B., Borer, J., and Sarapa, A.: The clinical pharmacology of antiarrhythmic drugs, part II. Cardiovasc. Nurs., 10:27-31, 1974.

Mayer, G. G., and Kaelin, P. B.: Arrhythmias and cardiac output. Am. J. Nurs., 72:1597-1600, 1972.

McAllister, R. G.: The possible role of anti-arrhythmic drugs in the prevention of sudden death. Heart Lung 2:857-861, 1973.

Rodman, M. J.: Drugs used in the CCU. R.N., 32:55-60, 1969.

Rodman, M. J.: Drugs used in cardiovascular disease. R. N., 36:55-56, 1973.

Shinn, A. F., Collins, D. N., and Hoops, E. J.: Drug interactions of common CCU medication. Am. J. Nurs., 74:1442-1446, 1974.

16

THE PATIENT WITH CONGESTIVE HEART FAILURE

TEXTBOOKS SUGGESTED FOR THIS STUDY

Asperheim, K., and Eisenhauer, L. A.: The Pharmacologic Basis of Patient Care, ed. 2. W. B. Saunders Co., Philadelphia, 1973, Chapters 3 and 19.

Bergersen, B.: Pharmacology in Nursing, ed. 13. C. V. Mosby Co., St. Louis, 1976, Chapters 10, 18, 19.

Brunner, L. S., and Suddarth, D. S.: Textbook of Medical-Surgical Nursing. J. B. Lippincott Co., Philadelphia, 1975, Chapters 17, 18, and 19.

Goodman, L., and Gilman, A. (eds.): The Pharmacological Basis of Therapeutics, ed. 5. Macmillan Co., New York, 1975, Chapters 12, 31, 32, 36, 39, 47, and 49.

Luckmann, J., and Sorensen, K.: Medical-Surgical Nursing—A Psychophysiologic Approach. W. B. Saunders Co., Philadelphia, 1974, Chapters 49, 50, and 51.

Rodman, M. J., and Smith, D. W.: Clinical Pharmacology in Nursing, J. B. Lippincott Co., Philadelphia, 1974, Chapters 27, 28, and 29.

Shafer, K., et al: Medical-Surgical Nursing, ed. 6. C. V. Mosby Co., St. Louis, 1975, Chapter 17.

PAST MEDICAL HISTORY

Frederick Peterson, a 66-year-old carpenter, was admitted to the hospital while on vacation. He began to develop signs and symptoms of fluid retention during the two weeks prior to admission. He had progressively increasing shortness of breath, three-pillow orthopnea, dyspnea on exertion, and paroxysmal noctural dyspnea with a six to seven pound weight gain during the past week. He has had four myocardial infarctions during the previous eight years and now has occasional episodes of angina. At the time of admission he was taking the following medications:

Digoxin (Lanoxin) 0.25 mg p.o. b.i.d.
Nitroglycerin (Nitrostat) 0.3 mg sublingual p.r.n.
Furosemide (Lasix) 40 mg p.o. b.i.d.

PRESENT HOSPITAL ADMISSION

First Hospital Day

7:00 P. M.—9:00 P.M. Mr. Peterson was admitted from the emergency room to the medical intensive care unit at 7:00 P. M. On admission he had a hacking cough, a few bibasilar rales, but was in no marked distress. His jugular veins were distended even when sitting; however, there was no cyanosis or edema of his extremities. His vital signs on admission were temperature 97.4° F., orally, radial pulse 46, apical pulse 92 and irregular, respirations 20, and blood pressure 100/60. His weight was 149½ pounds. The following diagnoses were made:

Congestive heart failure
Digoxin toxicity

Medical Orders

(1) Diet: 2 gm sodium, restrict fluids to 600 ml in 24 hours
(2) Serum potassium, serum sodium, serum chloride, and BUN stat.
(3) Daily serum potassium levels
(4) Bedrest on cardiac monitor
(5) Serum digoxin level in A. M.
(6) Diphenylhydantoin sodium (Dilantin) 100 mg IV now
(7) Atropine 0.5 mg IV p.r.n. for slow ventricular rate (less than 35 beats/minute)
(8) Lidocaine (Xylocaine) 50 mg IV bolus, then Xylocaine 1-4 mg IV drip for significant premature ventricular contractions (PVC's)
(9) Glyceryl guaiacolate (Robitussin) 10 ml p.o. for cough every 6 hours
(10) Dioctyl sodium sulfosuccinate (Colace) 100 mg p.o. b.i.d.

Study Questions

1. What factors in the medical history predispose Mr. Peterson to digoxin toxicity?

2. What are the signs and symptoms of digoxin toxicity? Which of these were noted on the first hospital day?

3. Mr. Peterson does not have any history of convulsions or other neurological disorders. Describe the use of diphenylhydantoin sodium (Dilantin) in the treatment of Mr. Peterson's heart disease. What nursing observations should be made to determine its effectiveness?

4. What is the action of atropine, a parasympatholytic agent, in the treatment of bradycardias?

5. What aspect of Mr. Peterson's cardiac problem does lidocaine affect?

6. How would you prepare and give a bolus of IV lidocaine?

7. Describe the physiological effects of glyceryl guaiacolate. Why is it ordered for a patient who has congestive heart failure? What instructions should be given to the patient before administering this medication to promote its demulcent action?

8. Why is dioctyl sodium sulfocuccinate (Colace) a desirable stool softener for patients with congestive heart failure?

9:00 P. M.—11:30 P. M. Mr. Peterson was lying comfortably in a semi-Fowler's position which made his breathing less labored; however, he continued to become dyspneic when he moved about in bed. The cardiac monitor showed atrial fibrillation with a slow ventricular response and PVC's in a bigeminal rhythm.

Laboratory Results

Blood urea nitrogen	23 mg/100 ml
Serum potassium	4.6 mEq/L
Serum sodium	133 mEq/L

11:30 P. M. Mr. Peterson's radial pulse was between 30 and 40 beats per minute and his apical pulse was between 70 and 80 beats per minute. His respirations were 30 per minute and he complained of shortness of breath. Jugular vein distension was present along with sacral edema and bibasilar rales.

Medical Orders

(1) Furosemide (Lasix) 40 mg IV stat.
(2) Add potassium chloride 30 mEq to 300 ml dextrose 5% in water to run at 50 ml per hour; then replace infusion with a heparin lock

Study Questions

9. What observations of Mr. Peterson's condition indicate that digoxin toxicity was still present?

10. Describe the signs and symptoms which indicate Mr. Peterson's need for IV furosemide (Lasix).

11. Describe the pathophysiology of fluid retention during congestive heart failure. How does furosemide alter this pathophysiology?

12. What changes in Mr. Peterson's condition would indicate the effectiveness of furosemide therapy?

13. What should the nurse tell Mr. Peterson to expect as a result of furosemide therapy?

14. What specific nursing observations must be made when a patient is on a potent diuretic?

15. Why were large doses of IV potassium chloride ordered for Mr. Peterson?

Second Hospital Day

7:00 A. M.—3:00 P. M. Mr. Peterson slept intermittently during the night and appeared less dyspneic at rest with respirations 24 per minute. Premature ventricular contractions (PVC's) in a bigeminal pattern still appeared which responded to lidocaine 50 mg given in an IV bolus. Mr. Peterson also continued to have a pulse deficit of 35 to 40 beats per minute. His weight at 7:00 A. M. was 145¾ pounds. His intake was 450 ml and his output was 700 ml for the previous 12 hours. Mr. Peterson stated that he felt more rested, although he appeared weak and was eating very slowly.

Laboratory Results

Serum potassium	4.8 mEq/L
Serum sodium	136 mEq/L
Serum chloride	92 mEq/L

Medical Orders

(1) Spironolactone (Aldactone) 50 mg p.o. b.i.d.
(2) Furosemide (Lasix) 40 mg IV stat.
(3) Serum potassium at 10:00 A. M.
(4) If serum potassium normal, give furosemide (Lasix) 80 mg IV at 11:00 A. M. and potassium chloride 20 mEq p.o.
(5) Serum potassium at 3:00 P. M.

3:00 P. M.—11:00 P. M. During the evening, Mr. Peterson began to feel a little better. The cardiac monitor showed only occasional PVC's with the basic rhythm still atrial fibrillation at 60 to 70 beats per minute. Serum potassium level at 3:00 P. M. was 5.0 mEq/L. At 8:00 P. M. the physician reevaluated Mr. Peterson's condition.

Medical Orders

(1) Mercaptomerin (Thiomerin) 1 ml IM now
(2) Flurazepam hydrochloride (Dalmane) 30 mg p.o. h.s. p.r.n.

Study Questions

16. Mr. Peterson was given spironolactone and furosemide. Describe the site of action of these two drugs and their effectiveness when administered together. How do their side effects differ?

17. When diuretic therapy is used, fluid and electrolyte disturbances are common. What is being done for Mr. Peterson to prevent this from occurring?

18. What nursing observations and actions are related to the potential fluid and electrolyte imbalances?

19. Describe how the nurse should carry out the medical order which reads, "If serum potassium normal, give furosemide (Lasix) 80 mg IV at 11:00 A. M. and potassium chloride 20 mEq p.o."

20. What type of medication is mercaptomerin? Which actions of this medication should be discussed by the nurse and Mr. Peterson?

21. Why was flurazepam hydrochloride ordered? What effect should it have for

Mr. Peterson?

Third Hospital Day

9:00 A. M.—12:00 M. Mr. Peterson's condition appeared generally improved. He had only an occasional cough and was not complaining of dyspnea. His lungs sounded clear to auscultation. He continued to have jugular vein distention but this was noted to be less severe. His heart rhythm remained unchanged with an irregular rate and a pulse deficit of 20 beats per minute. His early morning weight was 143¾ pounds, and his intake was 600 ml and output 1310 ml for the previous 24 hours.

<u>Laboratory Results</u>

Digoxin level	4.56 µg/ml
Serum potassium	5.1 mEq/L
Serum sodium	137 mEq/L
Serum chloride	95 mEq/L

<u>Medical Orders</u>

(1) Furosemide (Lasix) 80 mg p.o. b.i.d. today
(2) Repeat serum potassium at 3:00 P. M.

12:00 M.—6:00 P. M. Since Mr. Peterson's condition had stabilized, he was transferred to the intermediate care unit. At the time of transfer, he was noted to have sacral edema and mild pitting edema of his feet. His color was pale with no cyanosis. His skin was warm and dry, and he had no complaints of shortness of breath.

6:00 P. M.—11:00 P. M. Mr. Peterson's evening nurse reported to his physician that his urine output was between 100 and 120 ml every two hours. His color appeared a little cyanotic and he began to have periods of dyspnea on exertion. He was also complaining of nausea and ate very little dinner. The physician examined Mr. Peterson.

<u>Medical Orders</u>

(1) Oxygen 4 L per minute via nasal cannula
(2) Prochlorperazine (Compazine) 10 mg IM every 4 hours p.r.n. for nausea.
(3) Ethacrynic acid (Edecrin) 50 mg IV stat.
(4) Call physician if urine output falls below 250 ml/shift

Study Questions

22. Mr. Peterson's diagnosis of digoxin toxicity was confirmed by the reported serum digoxin level. What is considered a therapeutic serum digoxin level?

23. What is the relationship between Mr. Peterson's weight changes, intake and output record, and the diagnosis of digoxin toxicity?

24. What is the relationship between the action of digoxin and the serum potassium level? How can this relationship be affected by diuretic therapy?

25. When a patient is receiving digitalis therapy, potassium, and diuretics, what observations must be made by the nurses caring for the patient?

26. What type of medication is ethacrynic acid (Edecrin)? Why was it ordered stat. for Mr. Peterson? What is the site of action of this drug as compared to furosemide and spironolactone?

27. What is the significance of the doctor requesting to be notified of a drop in urine output?

28. Mr. Peterson was given prochlorperazine (Compazine) for nausea. What are some of the possible causes for nausea? Describe the action of prochlorperazine and discuss its other uses.

Fourth Hospital Day

6:00 A. M.—1:00 P. M. Mr. Peterson's condition remained the same during the night. His skin was warm and dry, sacral edema and marked neck vein distention were still present; and he slept with the bed in a semi-Fowler's position because of occasional dyspnea. His weight at 7:00 A. M. was 142 pounds, and his intake was 565 ml and output 1100 ml for the previous 24 hours. His heart rate was still irregular with atrial fibrillation and occasional PVC's. His radial pulse was 40 beats per minute and his apical pulse was 72 beats per minute.

Laboratory Results

Serum potassium	5.2 mEq/L
Serum sodium	139 mEq/L
Serum chloride	94 mEq/L

Medical Orders

(1) Ethacrynic acid (Edecrin) 50 mg IV this A. M.
(2) Diphenylhydantoin sodium (Dilantin) 150 mg IV and 150 mg IM stat.
(3) Obtain serum potassium at 3:00 P. M.

1:00 P. M.—7:00 P. M. Mr. Peterson's color improved and his oxygen was discontinued. He appeared more comfortable and stated that he felt much better this afternoon. His cardiac monitor pattern showed that he had only rare PVC's, and clinically his pulse deficit was decreasing.

7:00 P. M.—11:00 P. M. Mr. Peterson continued to feel better during the day. From 7:00 A. M. to 7:00 P. M. his intake was 550 ml and his output was 1195 ml. His 3:00 P. M. serum potassium was 4.3 mEq/L, and potassium chloride 20 mEq/L was administered orally. His heart rate continued in atrial fibrillation with only rare PVC's reported.

Study Questions

29. Considering Mr. Peterson's diagnosis of congestive heart failure, digoxin toxicity, and subsequent medication therapy, describe his clinical condition at 6:00 A. M. What nursing actions should be considered for a patient who has had this type of response to medication therapy?

30. Mr. Peterson's daily weights show a 7½ pound weight loss since admission. Discuss this weight loss considering his diuretic and daily intake and output record.

31. What changes are apparent in Mr. Peterson's condition at 1:00 P. M. and 7:00 P. M.? Consider the medications received at 9:00 A. M. when giving your answer.

32. Explain the change in Mr. Peterson's cardiac pattern in response to his medication therapy.

Summary of Hospitalization from Fifth to Twelfth Hospital Days

Mr. Peterson continued to diurese and by the twelfth hospital day he had lost a total of 23 pounds in weight. His neck vein distention was markedly decreased. His cardiac rhythm continued to improve with less ventricular irregularity and spontaneous conversion to normal sinus rhythm on the ninth day. At that time digoxin was ordered as follows:

(1) Digoxin (Lanoxin) 0.125 mg IV stat., then
(2) Digoxin (Lanoxin) 0.125 mg p.o. every day
(3) Get digoxin blood level after first digoxin dose

Mr. Peterson was discharged on the twelfth hospital day.

Discharge Orders

(1) Digoxin (Lanoxin) 0.125 mg p.o. every day
(2) Spironolactone with hydrochlorthiazide (Aldactazide) 1 tablet p.o. every day
(3) Low sodium diet
(4) Teach patient necessity of sodium and fluid restriction with a close eye on body weight
(5) Give patient his discharge summary for his own physician

Study Questions

33. What is the relationship between the conversion of Mr. Peterson's heart rhythm to a normal sinus rhythm and the subsequent order for digoxin to be administered intravenously?

34. How was the adequacy of Mr. Peterson's digoxin order evaluated?

35. Discuss Mr. Peterson's discharge medications considering the long term therapy for congestive heart failure.

36. Develop a teaching plan for Mr. Peterson. Include his discharge medications in the plan as well as the necessity of sodium and fluid restriction and the recording of body weights.

REFERENCES

Gans, J. A.: Digitalis glycosides, Nursing '73, 3:59-64, 1973.

Grollman, A.: How drugs work: diuretics, Consultant, 12:53-55, 1972.

King, J., et al.: Recent advances in therapy for refractory CHF, Geriatrics, 28:94-102, 1973.

Levitt, B., Borer, J., and Sarapa, A.: The clinical pharmacology of antiarrhythmic drugs, part I. Cardiovasc. Nurs., 10:23-26, 1974.

Rasmussen, S., et al.: The pharmacology and clinical use of digitalis. Cardiovasc. Nurs., 11:23-28, 1975.

Reed, G. M.: Confused about potassium? Nursing '74, 7:21-27, 1974.

Rodman, M. J.: Drugs used in cardiovascular disease. R. N., 36:55-56, 1973.

Sanderson, R. G., and Goldman, M. J.: Cardiac drugs. In Sanderson, R. G. (ed.): The cardiac patient. W. B. Saunders Co., Philadelphia, 1972, p. 316-345.

Schneider, S. J., and Boyce, B. A.: Complications of diuretic therapy. Am. J. Nurs., 68:1903-1907, September, 1968.

17

THE PATIENT WITH TUBERCULOSIS

TEXTBOOKS SUGGESTED FOR THIS STUDY

Asperheim, M. K., and Eisenhauer, L. A.: The Pharmacologic Basis of Patient Care, ed. 2., W. B. Saunders Co., 1973, Chapter 10.

Bergersen, B.: Pharmacology in Nursing, ed. 13. C. V. Mosby Co., St. Louis, 1976, Chapters 20 and 23.

Brunner, L. S., and Suddarth, D.: Textbook of Medical-Surgical Nursing, J. B. Lippincott Co., Philadelphia, 1975, Chapter 37.

Goodman, L., and Gilman, A., (eds.): The Pharmacological Basis of Therapeutics, ed. 5. Macmillan Co., New York, 1975, Chapters 10, 58, 60, and 71.

Luckmann, J., and Sorensen, K.: Medical-Surgical Nursing—A Psychophysiologic Approach, W. B. Saunders Co., Philadelphia, 1974, Chapter 71.

Rodman, M. J., and Smith, D.: Clinical Pharmacology in Nursing. J. B. Lippincott Co., Philadelphia, 1974, Chapter 42.

Shafer, K. N., et al: Medical Surgical Nursing, ed. 6. C. V. Mosby Co., St. Louis, 1975, Chapter 22.

PAST MEDICAL HISTORY

Mrs. Costales, a 45-year-old manager of a small waterfront hotel, has had a history of nonproductive cough for the past two months. After a month of ineffective home treatment with cough medicines, Mrs. Costales sought medical attention. The initial workup revealed additional symptoms of fatigue, generalized malaise, poor appetite, and epigastric pain. Diagnostic tests showed negative gallbladder and gastrointestinal series, and two strongly positive PPD's. A chest x-ray study showed a left-side infiltrate . A diagnosis of pneumonia was made. Treatment with ampicillin on an outpatient basis was begun. After two weeks a repeat chest x-ray film demonstrated no improvement of the left-sided infiltrate; in addition a thin-walled cyst with air-fluid level in the left apex was seen.

Mrs. Costales was admitted to the hospital with the diagnosis of lung abscess. Sputum specimens were ordered and antibiotic therapy continued. Although her cough persisted, Mrs. Costales denied symptoms of tuberculosis such as night sweats, weight loss, and chest pain. Treatment for the diagnosis of lung abscess continued for two weeks and was interrupted with the occurrence of three events: development of fever, an episode of hemoptysis, and a sputum culture positive for acid-fast bacteria. Mrs. Costales was immediately transferred to a municipal tuberculosis sanitarium with a diagnosis of pulmonary tuberculosis, active, cavitary.

PRESENT HOSPITAL ADMISSION

First Hospital Day

Mrs. Costales was admitted in no acute distress at 11:55 A.M, accompanied by her husband and daughter. She was described as a 62-inch, 124-pound well developed, well nourished, slightly obese female who did not smoke or drink alcoholic beverages. She denied any significant medical or surgical ailments. The physical examination was negative except for the lungs which were clear to percussion with some dullness at the left base, decreased breath sounds, and both inspiratory and expiratory rales and rhonchi in the left lung.

Medical Orders

(1) Regular diet
(2) Chest x-ray, postero-anterior and lateral
(3) Electrocardiogram
(4) Complete blood count
(5) VDRL
(6) Alkaline phosphatase, serum bilirubin, transaminase
(7) Fasting blood glucose and 2-hour post-prandial blood glucose following 100 gm carbohydrate meal
(8) 24-hour sputum collection for acid-fast bacteria, 6 specimens (by gastric aspiration if no sputum). If one of the first three specimens is positive for acid-fast bacteria, collect only three specimens.
(9) Tomogram of left lung
(10) Chloral hydrate (Noctec) 500 mg. h.s. p.r.n. for 3 nights

On admission Mrs. Costales' vital signs were temperature 98.4° F. orally, pulse 100, respirations 20, and blood pressure 102/70. At 12:30 P.M. she had an emesis of undigested food. She ate poorly and seemed to be in an angry and sullen mood. She complained about not receiving anything to eat or drink "at that other hospital" and complained at length about her family physician.

Vital Signs

3:00 P. M. Temperature 98.6° F. orally, pulse 88, respirations 18, blood pressure 100/80
8:00 P. M. Temperature 98.6° F. orally, pulse 100, respirations 20

Study Questions

1. Prior to her admission, Mrs. Costales had two strongly-positive PPD's. What does PPD mean? What classification of drug is PPD? By what other name may the PPD be called?

2. What is the immunologic significance of a positive PPD?

3. Describe the ways PPD is administered.

4. What problem may be associated with a subcutaneous administration of PPD?

5. How is a PPD recorded and how is it read?

6. Why is ampicillin, a broad-spectrum antibiotic, ineffective for tuberculosis? Relate the reason to the nature of the Mycobacterium.

Second Hospital Day

4:00 A. M. Mrs. Costales told the nurse that she vomited earlier during the night and had flushed it down the toilet. The bathroom had an odor of emesis. Mrs. Costales seemed pale, tired, and worn out. She was given a sandwich which she ate. Following this, she seemed to sleep better than earlier when she was observed to cough frequently. She expectorated small amounts of cloudy sputum with a few pale-yellow mucus plugs.

Vital Signs

6:00 A. M. Temperature 98.2°F., pulse 96, respirations 22, blood pressure 150/90

At 8:30 A. M. Mrs. Costales rather sadly kept asking the nurse why it had taken so long to find out what was wrong with her.

Laboratory Results

Chest x-ray	Large cavity at left apex approximately 6 cm. Perifocal infiltrates present
Sputum smear	Positive for acid-fast bacteria 20/100 fields
Urine smear	Negative

WBC - 10,700 per cu mm

(Differential)

Stabs	14%	Hemoglobin	10.8 gm/100 ml
Segs	60%		
Lymphocytes	21%	Hematocrit	36.0%
Monocytes	4%		
Eosinophils	1%		

Urinalysis	Specific Gravity	1.028
	Albumin	1+
	Sugar	3+
Chemistries	Bilirubin	
	Direct	0.1 mg/100 ml
	Indirect	0.3 mg/100 ml
	Total:	0.4 mg/100 ml
	SGOT	18 units
	SGPT	16 units
	Alkaline phosphatase	2.8 Bodansky units

Laboratory Results (Continued)

	Fasting blood glucose	424 mg/100 ml
	2 hr. post-prandial glucose	455 mg/100 ml
VRDL	Negative	
Electrocardiogram	Sinus tachycardia with atrial and ventricular rate of 110/minute	

On the basis of the urinalysis, fasting and post-prandial blood glucoses, the diagnosis of diabetes mellitus, adult onset, was made. During his visit, the physician spent time explaining the diagnosis of tuberculosis and diabetes to Mrs. Costales.

Medical Orders

(1) Testape q.i.d. a.c.
(2) Sliding scale regular insulin
    1+ = 5 units
    2+ = 10 units
    3+ = 15 units
    4+ = 20 units
(3) 1800 Calorie diabetic diet
(4) Elixir of terpin hydrate 10 ml every 4 hours p.r.n. for cough
(5) Streptomycin 1 gm daily IM
(6) Rifampin (Rifadin) 600 mg daily
(7) Ethambutol hydrochloride (Myambutol) 800 mg daily
(8) NPH insulin 15 units every A. M., start tomorrow A. M.

Vital Signs

8:00 P. M. Temperature 102.8° F., pulse 100, respirations 28, blood pressure 170/88

Medical Orders

Aspirin 600 mg every 4 hours p.r.n. for temperature over 102° F. orally

Mrs. Costales had stress incontinence with her coughing. She refused her cough medicine, stating she was allergic to it. After being questioned further, she stated she meant the cough medicine had not ever relieved her cough.

Vital Signs

10:00 P. M. Temperature 102° F., pulse 120, respirations 32

Study Questions

7. Discuss the reason for each of the blood chemistry tests and complete blood count ordered for Mrs. Costales as they relate to anticipated tuberculosis chemother-

apy.

8. Compare Mrs. Costales' prescribed medications to other drugs commonly used to treat tuberculosis.

9. What is the mode of action of antitubercular drugs?

10. List the dosage and the side and toxic effects of streptomycin.

11. What is the usual dosage of rifampin and its side and toxic effects?

12. What is the usual dosage of ethambutol and its side and toxic effects?

13. Compare the side and toxic effects of the drugs ordered for Mrs. Costales with the side and toxic effects of para-amino salicylic acid and isoniazid.

14. Discuss why the pharmacological treatment of tuberculosis includes more than one anti-tubercular drug.

15. What is the action of elixir of terpin hydrate? Why is it ordered for Mrs. Costales? What instructions should the nurse give Mrs. Costales when administering this medication?

16. What are the possible reasons for Mrs. Costales' vomiting on the second hospital day? Discuss nursing implications of her vomiting and their relationship to drug therapy.

17. What actions have been taken in the situation to deal with Mrs. Costales' vomiting?

Third Hospital Day

12:00 A. M.—6:00 A.M. Vital signs were temperature 99.8° F., pulse 96, respirations 20. Mrs. Costales had a moist productive cough and was expectorating into tissues. She perspired profusely. Elixir of terpin hydrate was taken at 12:15 A. M. Mrs. Costales continued to cough at intervals. Her sputum contained 10 ml of cloudy saliva, yellow sputum plugs, and one blood-streaked plug.

<u>Vital Signs</u>

6:00 A. M. Temperature 100° F., pulse 100, respirations 28, blood pressure 140/84
10:00 A. M. Temperature 98.8° F., pulse 118, respirations 24

<u>Laboratory Results</u>

Sputum smear Positive for acid-fast bacteria 20/100 fields

12:00 P. M.—3:00 P. M. Testape showed 1+ glucose in the urine. Regular insulin 5 units was given. Mrs. Costales seemed to be tolerating her medications well. Five ml of cloudy sputum with a small amount of dark-pink mucus was noted.

Vital Signs

3:00 P. M.	Temperature 99.2° F., pulse 114, respirations 22, blood pressure 148/90
8:00 P. M.	Temperature 100.8° F., pulse 104, respirations 22, blood pressure 140/80. Mrs. Costales expectorated a scant amount of mucus with dark-red streaking.
10:00 P. M.	Temperature 100.4° F., pulse 100, respirations 28

Fourth Hospital Day

6:00 A. M.—12:00 P. M. During the night Mrs. Costales produced 30 ml of sputum which was greenish-yellow with pink mucus plugs. She denied having any pain or discomfort and slept well most of the night. At 7:30 A. M. Mrs. Costales was up and ambulating. She had an occasional cough but stated that it had improved.

12:00 P. M.—4:00 P. M. Testape showed 2+ glucose in the urine. Regular insulin 10 units was given. Mrs. Costales was disappointed regarding the positive Testape reading. Explanation was given by the nurse regarding the reason for continued positive Testape and the time needed for diabetic regulation. At 3:00 P. M. Mrs. Costales was resting. She stated that she was tired and sore from the injections. Vital signs were: temperature 99° F., pulse 100, respirations 24, blood pressure 142/98.

Laboratory Results

Sputum smear	Negative

Fifth Hospital Day

6:00 A. M.—12:00 P. M. Vital signs were weight 127½ pounds, temperature 99.8° F., pulse 104, respirations 22, blood pressure 138/100. At 12:00 P. M. Testape showed 3+ glucose in the urine. Regular insulin 15 units was given. Mrs. Costales had a quiet and restful day and offered no complaints.

8:00 P. M.—10:00 P. M. Vital signs were temperature 101.4° F., pulse 120, respirations 24, blood pressure 160/100. Mrs. Costales was very concerned about her elevated temperature.

Study Questions

18. What is the significance of Mrs. Costales' temperature-pulse-respirations patterns since admission? What changes are expected in the pattern with drug therapy?

19. What indications are there at this time that drug therapy is effective?

20. What is the relationship between Mrs. Costales' coughing and sputum production and her underlying pathophysiology? How are these symptoms related to drug therapy?

21. What nursing problems are associated with unrelieved coughing in the tuberculosis patient?

22. To what extent can the patient expect cough relief from elixir of terpin hydrate?

23. What clarification is necessary regarding Mrs. Costales' complaints of soreness from the injections on the fourth hospital day?

24. What nursing measures related to streptomycin administration can help minimize discomfort?

25. What is the significance of the negative sputum smear on the fourth hospital day? How does this affect isolation procedures and antibiotic therapy?

26. Why is vision testing often done prior to tuberculosis chemotherapy?

27. When isoniazid is used in tuberculosis chemotherapy, pyridoxine is also administered. What is the reason for this?

Sixth Hospital Day

6:00 A. M.—10:00 A. M. Vital signs were 98.8°F., pulse 94, respirations 24, blood pressure 144/90. During the night Mrs. Costales produced about 30 ml of frothy and cloudy saliva with streaks of bright-red mucus. She stated she experienced epigastric discomfort during the night but she had no discomfort this morning. Urine specimen #2 was sent to the laboratory for acid-fast smear.

10:00 A. M.—8:00 P. M. Vital signs were temperature 97.2° F., pulse 88, respirations 20, blood pressure 120/80. Mrs. Costales was up and ambulating in her room. She stated she seemed to tire easily. She was encouraged to change to street clothes. Scant amount of sputum was present in the sputum cup. Mrs. Costales was eating very well.

Laboratory Results (10:00 A. M.)

Sputum smear	Negative
Urine smear	Negative

8:00 P. M.—10:00 P. M. Vital signs were temperature 99.2° F., pulse 100, respirations 24, blood pressure 130/84. A moderate amount of tan blood-streaked mucus was noted in the sputum cup.

Seventh Hospital Day

6:00 A. M.—12:00 P. M. Vital signs were temperature 99.2°F., pulse 90, respirations 28, blood pressure 144/86. Mrs. Costales expectorated approximately 10 ml greenish-brown mucus. Sputum specimen 6 was sent to the laboratory.

Laboratory Results

Sputum smear	Negative

12:00 P. M.—3:00 P. M. Vital signs were temperature 99° F., pulse 94, respirations 22, blood pressure 130/90. Mrs. Costales stated that she dreaded the injections she was receiving every day but did not resist them. Although she had been encouraged to wear street clothes, she continued to wear a hospital gown. She had done her own urine testing for glucose with Testape and read them accurately. At 12:00 P. M. the Testape showed 3+ glucose in the urine. Regular insulin 15 units was given.

Medical Orders

(1) Fasting blood glucose in A. M.
(2) 2-hour post-prandial blood glucose
(3) Ferrous sulfate (Feosol) 300 mg t.i.d. p.o.

Vital Signs

3:00 P. M. Temperature 99.4^{o} F., pulse 100, respirations 24, blood pressure 120/80
8:00 P. M. Temperature 100.2^{o} F., pulse 100, respirations 28, blood pressure 150/90. Mrs. Costales states she felt better and a little stronger.

Eighth Hospital Day

Vital Signs

6:00 A. M. Temperature 98° F., pulse 100, respirations 28, blood pressure 130/90

Laboratory Results

Fasting blood glucose	176 mg/100 ml
2-hour post-prandial glucose	129 mg/100 ml

12:00 P. M.—8:00 P. M. Testape showed 2+ glucose in the urine. Regular insulin 10 units was given. At 8:00 P. M. vital signs were temperature 98.6^{o} F., pulse 98, respirations 24, blood pressure 112/80. Mrs. Costales' coughing had subsided and there was scant sputum produced.

Medical Orders

NPH insulin 18 units daily, IM, start tomorrow A. M.

Fourteenth Hospital Day

Mrs. Costales had remained afebrile and her cough had disappeared. Her weight was 128 pounds. The diabetes was now controlled with NPH 18 units daily. She has been involved in occupational therapy. She stated that since she no longer coughs and does not have a fever, the injections and other medications will soon stop.

28. What is the pattern of Testape results requiring coverage with regular insulin on the 3rd, 4th, 5th, and 7th hospital days?

29. How might this pattern of positive Testape results relate to the duration and peak action of NPH insulin?

30. Discuss the reason for the change in the NPH insulin order on the 8th hospital day.

31. What is the reason for the ferrous sulfate order on the 7th hospital day?

32. How would the nurse assess the effects of ferrous sulfate? What side effects should the nurse be watching for when administering ferrous sulfate?

33. What is the meaning of the fasting blood glucose and 2-hour post-prandial blood glucose on the 8th hospital day as they relate to pharmacological management of Mrs. Costales' diabetes?

34. What is the usual or recommended length of chemotherapy for tuberculosis?

35. Based on Mrs. Costales' comment on the 14th hospital day, discuss what patient teaching is needed.

36. The new anti-tubercular drugs have changed treatment of tuberculosis so that successful treatment is dependent on the patient's continuing to take his medication for a long time. What nursing actions are essential in helping these patients in this aspect of their care?

37. Describe follow-up necessary with Mrs. Costales' family and other contacts. What chemotherapeutic preventive measures are usually employed?

38. When Mrs. Costales is discharged, what specific aspects of patient teaching need reemphasis and introduction?

39. BCG is a tuberculosis vaccine. What are the indications for its use? How is it administered?

REFERENCES

American Lung Association. Diagnostic Standards and Classification of Tuberculosis and other Mycobacterial Diseases, New York, 1974.

American Lung Association. Introduction to Lung Disease, New York, 1973, pp. 34-48.

American Lung Association. The Tuberculin Skin Test, New York, 1974.

Clark, M. A.: Recent trends in tuberculosis care. Nurs. Clin. N. A., 9:157-164, 1974.

Clemens, J. H.: Tuberculosis: chemoprophylaxis and treatment. Postgrad. Med., 58:97-101, 1975.

Pitts, F. W.: Tuberculosis in Virginia. V. Med. Monthly, 11:1175-1179, 1972.

Radner, D. B.: Changing concepts in treatment of tuberculosis. Chest 61:520-523, 1973.

Robinson, A. M.: Pulmonary TB—not quite a disease of the past. R. N. 38:77-82, 1975.

18

THE PATIENT WITH CHRONIC OBSTRUCTIVE LUNG DISEASE

TEXTBOOKS SUGGESTED FOR THIS STUDY

Asperheim, M. K., and Eisenhauer, L. A.: The Pharmacologic Basis of Patient Care, ed. 2. W. B. Saunders Co., Philadelphia, 1973, Chapters 9, 12, 13, 15, 16, 17, and 19.

Bergersen, B.: Pharmacology in Nursing, ed. 13. C. V. Mosby Co., St. Louis, 1976, Chapters 10, 16, and 19.

Brunner, L. S., and Suddarth, D.: Textbook of Medical-Surgical Nursing, ed. 3. J. B. Lippincott Co., Philadelphia, 1974, Chapters 19, 25, and 27.

Shafer, K. N., et al: Medical Surgical Nursing, ed. 6. C. V. Mosby Co., St. Louis, 1975, Chapter 22.

PAST MEDICAL HISTORY

Edward Fernandez, a 67-year-old retired bricklayer, has had a long history of respiratory problems. Thirteen years ago he first visited a physician complaining of shortness of breath. Since that time he has had a downward battle with dyspnea, decreased exercise tolerance, and chronic cough. Several bouts of pneumonia and pulmonary infections have occurred, and Mr. Fernandez finally quit work five years ago because of his dyspnea. He has been unable to walk a flight of stairs, to eat an entire meal without having to stop because of shortness of breath, and to walk from one room to another without stopping to rest. Prior to his retirement, Mr. Fernandez was a heavy smoker and drinker. The medical regimen outlined by his physician since retirement included theophylline, ephedrine hydrochloride, phenobarbital (Tedral) 1 tablet four times a day and intermittent positive pressure breathing (IPPB) once a day as needed with isoetharine hydrochloride and phenylephrine hydrochloride (Bronkosol) and acetylcysteine (Mucomyst).

In addition to his pulmonary problems, Mr. Fernandez has had a history of epigastric distress, which has been treated with diet and antacids. In his most recent hospitalization six months ago, diagnostic tests confirmed right ventricular hypertrophy.

PRESENT HOSPITAL ADMISSION

First Hospital Day

Mr. Fernandez, accompanied by his wife, was admitted at 10:00 A. M. to the fourth floor of the medical center. During his admission physical examination, he said that he had swelling of his ankles for several weeks and was unable to lie down without becoming very short of breath. He was coughing up thick yellow mucus and could not walk from room to room. His wife stated that she would find him standing in one place bending over a table in order to breathe. At the time of admission he was noted to have a severe cough, chest discomfort, circumoral cyanosis and used his accessory muscles to breathe. He complained of occasional palpitations and frequently awakened at night unable to breathe. On admission his vital signs were blood pressure 138/86, pulse 86 and slightly irregular, respirations 42, temperature 100.8° F., and weight 153 pounds. The following diagnoses were made:

(1) Chronic obstructive pulmonary disease, probable silicosis with chronic bronchitis and emphysema
(2) Cor pulmonale secondary to pulmonary emphysema
(3) Acute upper respiratory infection
(4) Peptic ulcer disease by history

Medical Orders

(1) Digoxin (Lanoxin) 1.0 mg p.o. stat.
(2) Digoxin (Lanoxin) 0.5 mg p.o. in 6 hours
Digoxin (Lanoxin) 0.5 mg p.o. in 12 hours
Then give digoxin (Lanoxin) 0.25 mg p.o. every day
(2) Intermittent positive pressure breathing (IPPB) every 4 hours with isotharine hydrochloride and phenylephrine hydrochloride (Bronkosol) 0.5 ml
acetylcysteine (Mucomyst) 3.0 ml
(3) Furosemide (Lasix) 20 mg every A. M. p.o.
(4) Ampicillin (Polycillin) 500 mg IV per metriset every 6 hours
(5) Magnesium hydroxide and aluminum hydroxide (Maalox) 30 ml p.o. t.i.d.
(6) Cardiac monitor
(7) Lidocaine hydrochloride (Xylocaine) IV p.r.n. for significant premature ventricular contractions (PVC's)
(8) Serum potassium stat.

Study Questions

1. The primary purpose for therapy with digitalis glycosides is the treatment of congestive heart failure. Considering this fact, why did the physician order digoxin for Mr. Fernandez?

2. What is the purpose of the digoxin order as it is written?

3. Digitalis has positive inotropic, negative chronotropic, and negative dromotro-

phic effects on the heart. Which of Mr. Fernandez's signs and symptoms should be relieved by these actions? Why?

4. What nursing actions should be taken prior to the administration of digoxin? Why should such action be taken?

5. Toxic reactions to digitalis therapy commonly occur. What toxic effects must the nurse caring for Mr. Fernandez watch for and report? Include changes in cardiac rate, rhythm, and conduction in your answer.

6. IPPB has been ordered for Mr. Fernandez. Compare the reason it is used in the treatment of emphysema to its use in the treatment of pulmonary edema.

7. What are the nurse's responsibilities when an IPPB treatment is being administered?

8. What physiological responses will Mr. Fernandez have to the medication, Mucomyst and bronkosol, used during IPPB treatment?

9. Explain the reason furosemide was ordered for Mr. Fernandez. What is its action on the kidney? What is the body's physiological response?

10. When a patient is taking furosemide, what specific nursing observations must be made to determine drug effectiveness? What nursing observations must be made to determine side effects and toxic effects?

11. Why was Maalox ordered for Mr. Fernandez? What instructions should be given to the patient when administering this medication?

12. What type of antibiotic is ampicillin? For what types of diseases is it most useful? Why was it ordered for Mr. Fernandez?

1:00 P. M. Frequent multifocal PVC's were seen on the cardiac monitor and lidocaine was administered with immediate suppression of ectopic beats.

Study Questions

13. Why was lidocaine, a local anesthetic, ordered for control of PVC's?

14. What is the significance of the electrocardiogram tracing following the administration of lidocaine?

15. What is the relationship between the action of lidocaine, the electrocardiogram tracing, and the suppression of ectopic beats?

2:00 P. M.—5:30 P. M. The initial IPPB treatment with Bronkosol and Mucomyst was given. Mr. Fernandez tolerated it poorly. He complained that the medications made him nauseated and stood hunched over his bedside table while having the treatment. Laboratory results indicated that the serum potassium was 4.2 mEq/L. By

5:30 P. M. the physician had returned to the unit to reevaluate Mr. Fernandez's response to the initial treatments.

Medical Orders

(1) May use normal saline in IPPB if patient cannot tolerate the combination of isoetharine hydrochloride and phenylephrine hydrochloride (Bronkosol), and acetylcysteine (Mucomyst)
(2) Intravenous dextrose 5% in 0.2% sodium chloride solution with 15 mEq potassium chloride run at 75 ml/hour
(3) Saturated solution of potassium iodide 10 drops with juice t.i.d.
(4) Oxygen via nasal cannula 2-4 l p.r.n.
(5) Theophylline ethylenediamine (aminophylline) 250 mg i.v. in metriset to run over 20 minutes stat., then every 6 hours p.r.n. for severe dyspnea

6:00 P.M. IPPB treatment with normal saline was tolerated well and Mr. Fernandez stated "I feel a little better after this treatment." The theophylline was given i.v. without much relief. Vital signs were blood pressure 138/84, pulse 88, and respirations 44 and regular.

Study Questions

16. What is the relationship between the occurrence of nausea and the use of Bronkosol and Mucomyst for IPPB?

17. What effect will the IPPB treatments have using normal saline solution instead of Bronkosol and Mucomyst?

18. Why was potassium added to Mr. Fernandez' intravenous dextrose solution when the serum potassium was within normal limits?

19. What type of medication is saturated solution of potassium iodide? Why was it ordered for Mr. Fernandez? Why must it be given in juice?

20. What effect does theophylline have on the respiratory system? What complications might occur if it is given over a period shorter than twenty minutes?

21. Describe the nurse's responsibilities when administering a medication by intermittent intravenous infusion.

22. Discuss the medicolegal aspects of administering medications intravenously. How does the Nurse Practice Act define the nurse's responsibilities in this area?

Second Hospital Day

7:00 A.M. Vital signs were blood pressure 138/84, pulse 78 and regular, respirations 46 and regular. The night nurse reported that Mr. Fernandez had been hunched over his bedside table since 2:00 A.M. and stated that he was too tired for his 6:00 A.M. IPPB treatment. He refused his morning care and IPPB and was reported to have stood at his bedside all day. His feet were edematous, he was short of breath, and his skin was pale and moist.

Medical Orders

Theophylline, ephedrine hydrochloride, and phenobarbital (Tedral) 1 tablet p.o. every 6 hours p.r.n. for dyspnea

3:00 P.M.—11:00 P.M. Mr. Fernandez continued to refuse his IPPB treatments; however, he would take his other medications. When he was not leaning over his bedside table he would kneel on his bed hunched over a pillow with his knees drawn up to his chest, an unusual but comfortable position for Mr. Fernandez. His oxygen was running at 4 l and his lungs sounded congested with no expectoration. Mr. Fernandez had a severe episode of dyspnea at 7:00 P.M. and was given Tedral 1 tablet. Within twenty minutes the dyspnea had decreased and he was able to lie comfortably in a high Fowler's position.

Study Questions

23. Discuss Mr. Fernandez' physical symptoms on the second hospital day in relationship to his response to furosemide and theophylline.

24. Mr. Fernandez continued to refuse IPPB therapy. What nursing actions were appropriate at this time?

25. What is the therapeutic action of Tedral?

Third Hospital Day

7:00 A.M. Vital signs were blood pressure 130/80, pulse 68, and respirations 44. Mr. Fernandez received aminophylline 500 mg intravenously and Tedral 1 tablet p.o. at 6:00 A.M. with little relief. He still complained of wheezing and had several loose stools which kept him awake most of the night.

Laboratory Results

Digitalis blood levels in a high therapeutic range
Sputum culture showed normal throat flora with no pathogenic growth

Medical Orders

(1) Discontinue theophylline ethylenediamine (aminophylline)
(2) Hydrocortisone sodium succinate (Solu-Cortef) 200 mg i.v. per metriset every 6 hours
(3) Diazepam (Valium) 5 mg p.o. every 4 hours p.r.n.
(4) Discontinue magnesium hydroxide and aluminum hydrozide (Maalox)
(5) Aluminum hydroxide, magnesium hydroxide, and simethicone (Mylanta) 30 ml t.i.d. every 4 hours while awake

3:00 P.M. Mr. Fernandez refused treatment most of the morning. Bibasilar coarse rales were noted. By afternoon Mr. Fernandez was asleep but was noted to by dyspneic with a respiratory rate of 40/minute.

Study Questions

26. What are the possible causes of Mr. Fernandez' continued wheezing?

27. Is there any relationship between the physicians's decision to discontinue theophylline and order hydrocortisone?

28. A frequent side effect of cortisone therapy is sodium and water retention and potassium excretion. How might these adverse actions affect Mr. Fernandez' condition?

29. During Mr. Fernandez' first three hospital days, what changes in cardiac status can be attributed to the effects of digoxin?

30. What nursing actions could have been taken to make Mr. Fernandez more comfortable during the morning?

31. What change in Mr. Fernandez' condition occurred at 7:00 A.M. indicating the necessity for the orders to discontinue Maalox and administer Mylanta?

11:00 P.M. Physical examination of Mr. Fernandez revealed dyspnea, pitting edema of the ankles, and cold extremities. Mr. Fernandez continued to refuse IPPB treatment and complained of nausea after receiving ampicillin. Although he stood by his bed all evening, he was noted to be sleeping at 10:45 P.M. after receiving diazepam 5 mg p.o.

Study Questions

32. Discuss Mr. Fernandez' persistent dyspnea, edema, and cool extremities, considering his diagnosis and the medications he has been given to treat these signs and symptoms.

33. Has Mr. Fernandez shown any evidence of drug toxicity?

34. What type of medication is diazepam? Why was it ordered for Mr. Fernandez?

35. Mr. Fernandez has been receiving furosemide 20 mg every A.M. Why was he given an additional 40 mg at 11:00 P.M.?

Fourth Hospital Day

Vital signs were blood pressure 134/82, pulse 58, respirations 44, and weight 148 pounds. Mr. Fernandez spent a more comfortable night. He was able to lie flat in bed and was reported to have been dozing part of the night. He had no further bouts of nausea and accepted his IPPB treatment following which he expectorated a moderate amount of tenacious mucus. The morning Digoxin was held because his apical pulse was 48. He felt better as the day progressed with only a small amount of ankle edema noted.

Medical Orders

(1) Withhold digoxin (Lanoxin) today
(2) Starting in A.M. digoxin (Lanoxin) 0.125 mg p.o. every day

Study Questions

36. Discuss Mr. Fernandez' weight loss and decrease in edema in relationship to his medical therapy.

37. Explain the cause of his tenacious mucus and describe how and why it was expectorated following IPPB treatment.

38. Discuss the relationship of Mr. Fernandez' pulse rate and the adjustment of his digoxin dosage.

Fifth to Seventh Hospital Days

Mr. Fernandez' blood pressure remained within normal range, and his pulse ranged from 68 to 74 and remained regular. His lungs began to clear and he was able to lie down and sleep for several hours during the night. However, his weight began to rise and his urinary output decreased. He was maintained on the same medical regimen with the exception of hydrocortisone which was changed to 200 mg IV every 24 hours.

Study Questions

39. What is the relationship between Mr. Fernandez' increasing weight and decrease in urine output? What are the nursing responsibilities when this occurs?

40. Discuss the change in Mr. Fernandez' hydrocortisone order from 200 mg IV every 6 hours to 200 mg IV every 24 hours.

Progress Report

Mr. Fernandez' weight stabilized at 152 pounds, and he continued to improve. Hydrocortisone was discontinued and he was placed on prednisone 5 mg b.i.d. on the ninth hospital day. Although his lungs were improving, he had mild complaints of epigastric distress which was relieved by Mylanta. Episodic periods of mild dyspnea were relieved with Tedral. By the thirteenth hospital day, his prednisone was reduced to 5 mg p.o. every day and plans to discharge him were made.

Discharge Orders

(1) Prednisone 2.5 mg every day
(2) Theophylline, ephedrine hydrochloride, and phenobarbital (tedral) 1 tablet every 6 hours p.r.n. dyspnea

(3) Furosemide (Lasix) 20 mg p.o. every day
(4) Digoxin (Lanoxin) 0.125 mg p.o. every day
(5) IPPB daily as needed with:
isoetharine hydrochloride and phenylephrine hydrochloride (Bronkosol)
acetylcysteine (Mucomyst)
(6) Aluminum hydroxide, magnesium hydroxide, and simethicone (Mylanta)
30 ml p.o. q.i.d. between meals

Study Questions

41. Why is Mr. Fernandez' prednisone being decreased gradually rather than discontinued all at once?

42. There are many side effects of steriod therapy. What should Mr. Fernandez be told about them?

43. How can the nurse assist Mr. Fernandez and his family in obtaining an IPPB machine?

44. How should the nurse explain the importance of the order for Mylanta to Mr. Fernandez and his wife?

45. How can the daily administration of furosemide influence the occurrence of digoxin toxicity?

46. What is the relationship between the diet intake and the prevention of digoxin toxicity?

47. Develop a plan to help Mr. Fernandez take his medicatons at home. Plan a way to help him to remember what each medication is and at what time of day it should be taken.

REFERENCES

Blancher, G. C.: Caring for the patient with advanced emphysema, R.N. 37:41-42+, 1974.

Blount, M., et al.: Chronic steriod therapy. Am. J. Nurs., 74:1626-1631, 1974.

Ciuca, R.: Cor pulmonale. Nursing '73, 3:3-10+, 1973.

Cupit, C., et al.: Antacids. Am. J. Nurs., 72:2210-2212, 1972.

Fuhs, M., and Stein, A.: Better ways to cope with COPD. Nursing '76, 6:28-38, 1976.

Rasmussen, S., et al.: The pharmacology and clinical use of digitalis. Cardiovasc. Nurs., 11:23-28, 1975.

Rodman, M. J.: Drugs for acute respiratory failure. R.N. 38:49-56, 1975.

Rodman, M. J.: Drugs for allergic disorders. R.N. 34:63-69, 1971.

Rodman, M. J.: Drugs used against chronic airway obstruction. R.N. 37:45-55, 1974.

Winslow, E. H.: Digitalis. Am. J. Nurs., 74:1062-1065, 1974.

19

THE PATIENT WITH BURNS

TEXTBOOKS SUGGESTED FOR THIS STUDY

Asperheim, M. K., and Eisenhauer, L. A.: The Pharmacologic Basis of Patient Care, ed. 2. W. B. Saunders Co., Philadelphia, 1973, Chapters 18 and 19.

Bergersen, B.: Pharmacology in Nursing, ed. 13. C. V. Mosby Co., St. Louis, 1976, Chapter 18.

Brunner, L. S., and Suddarth, D.: Textbook of Medical Surgical Nursing, ed. 3. J.B. Lippincott Co., Philadelphia, 1975, Chapter 30.

Goodman, L., and Gilman, A. (eds.): The Pharmacological Basis of Therapeutics, ed. 5. Macmillan Co., New York, 1975, Chapters 10, 15, 36, 37, 48, 50, 56, 57, 58, 73, and 74.

Luckmann, J., and Sorensen, K.: Medical-Surgical Nursing — A Psychophysiologic Approach. W. B. Saunders Co., Philadelphia, 1974, Chapter 92.

Rodman, M. J., and Smith, D.: Pharmacology and Drug Therapy in Nursing. J. B. Lippincott Co., Philadelphia, 1968, Chapters 9, 43, and 45.

Shafer, K. N., et al.: Medical Surgical Nursing, ed. 6. C. V. Mosby Co., St. Louis, 1975, Chapter 29.

PRESENT HOSPITAL ADMISSION

Mr. Chang, a 43-year-old electrician, was admitted to the medical center at 3:45 P.M. with first degree burns of his face and ears and second degree burns of both lower arms and hands, anterior thighs and buttocks, sustained from an electrical flash fire. The fire occurred at about 2:30 P.M. His burns totaled approximately 35 per cent of his body surface. Mr. Chang weighs 160 pounds and is 67 inches tall. He attempted to extinguish the flames on his clothing by rolling on the ground outside the shed where the fire occurred.

This is Mr. Chang's first hospital admission and his medical history is essentially negative for cardiovascular, respiratory, and renal diseases, and diabetes mellitus. He has no known drug allergies and has not had a tetanus booster for 5 years.

First Hospital Day

Medical Orders (3:45 P.M.)

(1) Morphine sulfate 10 mg IV stat.

(2) Morphine sulfate 10 mg every 3-4 hours p.r.n. for pain IV
(3) Tetanus toxoid 0.5 ml IV stat.
(4) Silver sulfadiazine (Silvadene Cream) to all burned areas
(5) Neomycin sulfate and dexamethasone (NeoDECADRON Ophthalmic Solution) 2 drops in each eye q.i.d.
(6) Stat. laboratory tests: hemoglobin, hematocrit, urinalysis, serum sodium, potassium, chloride, urea nitrogen, carbon dioxide, glucose, total proteins, calcium, alkaline phosphatase, bilirubin, cholesterol, SGOT, serum osmolality
(7) Repeat serum sodium, potassium, chloride, urea nitrogen, carbon dioxide, and glucose at 8:00 A.M. and daily
(8) Repeat hemoglobin and hematocrit daily
(9) Repeat serum osmolality every 8 hours times three
(10) Intake and output — record hourly on flow sheet
(11) Foley catheter stat. to continuous drainage with urometer
(12) Monitor urine output hourly and notify physician if output falls below 50 ml/hour
(13) Vital signs every 15 minutes — record hourly on flow sheet
(14) Central venous pressure (CVP) hourly
(15) Reverse isolation
(16) Tracheostomy set at bedside
(17) Regulate room temperature at 85-88° F.
(18) NPO
(19) Intravenous fluids as follows:

<u>4:00 P.M. — 12:00 A.M.</u>

Left ankle — 1000 ml lactated Ringer's solution
500 ml 5% glucose in water

CVP line — 1000 ml lactated Ringer's solution
500 ml 5% glucose in water

Regulate each IV to run at 180 ml/hour

<u>12:00 A.M. — 8:00 A.M.</u>

Left ankle — 500 ml 5% glucose in water at 65 ml/hour

CVP line — 1000 ml lactated Ringer's solution at 125 ml/hour

<u>8:00 A.M. — 4:00 P.M.</u>

Left ankle — 500 ml 5% glucose in water at 65 ml/hour
CVP line — 1000 ml lactated Ringer's solution at 125 ml/hour

(20) Add aqueous penicillin 1 million units to each liter of IV fluid

4:00 P.M. In the emergency room, a CVP line was established via the right subclavian vein, and a cutdown was started in the left ankle with lactated Ringer's solution. Mr. Chang was awake, oriented in three spheres, and when questioned, stated he was in pain. He grimaced when the silver sulfadiazine cream was applied to the burned areas and when he was turned. However, he did not complain overtly of pain. Morphine sulfate 10 mg was administered IV at 4:00 P.M. Blood and urine specimens were obtained and sent to the laboratory for analysis. Hourly intake and output with vital signs were recorded on a burn flow sheet.

5:00 P.M. Mr. Chang was transferred from the emergency room to the intensive care unit and placed on a circo-electric bed.

Laboratory Results

Serum sodium	144 mEq/L
Serum potassium	3.3 mEq/L
Serum chloride	105 mEq/L
Serum carbon dioxide	24 mEq/L
Blood urea nitrogen	21 mg/100 ml
Serum glucose	155 mg/100 ml
Serum total protein	6.4 gm/100 ml
Serum calcium	9.0 mg/100 ml
Serum alkaline phosphatase	45 Bodansky units
Serum bilirubin	2.1 mg/100 ml
Serum cholesterol	200 mg/100 ml
Serum SGOT	28 units
Serum hemoglobin	16.1 gm/100 ml
Serum hematocrit	48.3%
Serum osmolality	310 mOs/kg

6:00 P.M. Mr. Chang was encouraged to cough and deep breathe every hour and was turned every two hours. His arms were elevated on pillows. His face and ears were swollen; his arms, hands, and thighs were "weeping" serous fluid. Silver sulfadiazine cream was reapplied where it had been washed off by the serous fluid.

Medical Orders

Add potassium chloride 20 mEq to current bottle of lactated Ringer's solution and another 20 mEq to the next 1000 ml of lactated Ringer's solution

8:00 P.M. Mr. Chang was given morphine 10 mg IV

Medical Orders

Salt-poor serum albumin (Albumisol) 200 ml IV stat.

11:30 P.M. The salt-poor albumin administration was completed. Mr. Chang was sleeping. There was no respiratory difficulty noted. Burned areas were "weeping" copious serous fluid.

11:45 P.M. 24-Hour Intake and Output

Intake: 2880 ml IV Output: 460 ml

FLOW SHEET — FIRST HOSPITAL DAY

Time	Temp	Pulse	Resp	BP	CVP	IV # 1 *	IV # 2 *	Output
4 P.M.	99	114	26					
5 P.M.		110	24	106/60	7.5	180 ml	180 ml	60 ml
6 P.M.	99	118	24	102/64	7.0	180 ml	180 ml	75 ml
7 P.M.		116	24	104/58	7.0	180 ml	180 ml	60 ml
8 P.M.	99.2	114	24	108/62	6.0	180 ml	180 ml	55 ml
9 P.M.		118	24	100/58	5.5	180 ml	180 ml	55 ml
10 P.M.	99.2	136	26	86/50	4.0	180 ml	180 ml	45 ml
11 P.M.		120	24	100/68	5.0	180 ml	180 ml	50 ml
12 A.M.	99.2	112	22	116/62	7.0	180 ml	180 ml	60 ml

* IV Intake # 1 = Left ankle * IV Intake # 2 = CVP

Study Questions

1. Why is it necessary to adequately control Mr. Chang's pain in the immediate postburn period? What is the potential effect of the untreated pain at this time? What cues should the nurse observe related to untreated pain?

2. What cultural aspects should the nurse consider in the evaluation of Mr. Chang's need for pain medication?

3. Relate the 4:00 P.M. vital signs (see FLOW CHART — FIRST HOSPITAL DAY) to the nursing evaluation of Mr. Chang's pain response. What indications are there that the morphine administered at 4:00 P.M. was effective?

4. What is the underlying pathophysiology of burns which makes it dangerous to give narcotic analgesics subcutaneously or intramuscularly in the immediate postburn period? Describe the toxic and side effects of morphine sulfate. What precautions are necessary to prevent side effects when the nurse administers IV morphine?

5. Discuss the reason for tetanus toxoid administration to Mr. Chang. Under what circumstances would tetanus antitoxin be given instead of tetanus toxoid? Describe the differences in relation to the immune response.

6. Prior to administration of aqueous penicillin, what history is necessary for safety? What side or toxic effects will application of this information prevent?

7. Discuss the range of effectiveness of aqueous penicillin and the rationale for intravenous aqueous penicillin administration.

8. What is the range of effectiveness for silver sulfadiazine? Compare this range with the three other major topical antibacterials used in burn management: mafenide acetate (Sulfamylon Cream), silver nitrate 0.5% solution, and gentamicin sulfate (Garamycin).

9. Compare the advantages and disadvantages of silver sulfadiazine to the other major drugs used for burn wounds. What side and toxic effects result from silver sulfadiazine?

10. Discuss the mode of application of silver sulfadiazine cream to Mr. Chang's burned areas for maximum effectiveness. How often does the nurse reapply this medication?

11. What is the rationale for the use of a topical antibacterial such as silver sulfadiazine when Mr. Chang is receiving a million units of aqueous penicillin intravenously with each liter of intravenous fluid?

12. How should the effectiveness of silver sulfadiazine and the aqueous penicillin be assessed?

13. Which pharmacological approach to burn wound management best minimizes the heat loss associated with the hypermetabolic state in the severly burned patient?

Why?

14. What is the action of neomycin sulfate and dexamethasone? How does this action differ from the administration of neomycin sulfate alone? Why is this combination indicated for Mr. Chang? What related nursing observations and actions are indicated for evaluating the effectiveness of the neomycin sulfate and dexamethasone?

15. The exact time when burns occur is important in planning care. What aspects of burn management requires knowledge of when burns were sustained?

16. Relate the schedule and amounts of fluid replacement in the first 24 hours to burn pathophysiology.

17. What clinical complications of burns are related to inadequate fluid administration? Describe the mechanism leading to these complications.

18. How should the nurse set up and mark the intravenous fluid bottles?

19. Which aspects of nursing assessment determine adequacy of fluid replacement for Mr. Chang?

20. Why is lactated Ringer's solution given during this time in such large amounts relative to glucose solution? What does lactated Ringer's solution contain?

21. What is the danger in the immediate postburn period of administration of large amounts of glucose solution IV or of giving Mr. Chang tap water by mouth? What are the signs and symptoms of the complications which occur with overtreatment with glucose in water?

22. Discuss the significance of Mr. Chang's CVP and vital signs at 10:00 P.M. Relate this to the order for salt-poor albumin.

23. What type of solution is salt-poor albumin? What physiologic function does it serve? Relate the need for salt-poor albumin to the pathophysiology of burns.

24. What are the pros and cons for the administration of colloid solution during the first 24 hours following burns? Give examples of colloid solutions which may be used.

25. What are the observable effects of salt-poor albumin therapy at 11:45 P.M.?

26. What is the basis for the 6:00 P.M. order for potassium chloride administration? Discuss potassium metabolism in the postburn period.

27. What precautions are necessary when the nurse administers potassium chloride intravenously to Mr. Chang? Describe the signs and symptoms of potassium deficits and excesses.

28. What is the rationale for reverse isolation as it is related to Mr. Chang's drug therapy?

29. Insulin has been used by some physicians in the treatment of severe burns. Relate the use of insulin to the metabolic disorder in burn pathophysiology.

30. What laboratory evidence is there that may support the use of insulin in Mr. Chang's burn management?

31. Which other physician's order at 3:45 P.M. on the first hospital day was directed toward minimizing heat loss and the metabolic disorder which occurs with severe burns?

Second Hospital Day

(See FLOW SHEET — SECOND HOSPITAL DAY for vital signs, CVP, intake and output)

Laboratory Results (1:00 A.M.)

Serum osmolality	306 mOs/kg

1:00 A.M. Mr. Chang was awake and restless. Silver sulfadiazine was reapplied to thighs, arms, and hands. Mr. Chang grimaced and stated he was uncomfortable. Morphine 10 mg was given. He continued to be restless throughout the rest of the night.

Medical Orders (8:00 A.M.)

Acetaminophen (Tylenol) suppository 600 mg every 3-4 hours p.r.n. for temperature of 101° F. orally and over

9:00 A.M. Silver sulfadiazine was reapplied to burned areas as necessary. Wounds were weeping copious amounts of serous fluid. Mr. Chang appeared comfortable. Morphine 10 mg was given.

9:30 A.M. Mr. Chang complained of nausea but did not vomit.

Medical Orders (10:00 A.M.)

(1) Vital signs every hour, and CVP every 4 hours
(2) Continue to measure urine output every hour
(3) Discontinue morphines
(4) Meperidine hydrochloride (Demerol) 50 mg / Promethazine hydrochloride (Phenergan) 25 mg — IM every 3-4 hours p.r.n. for pain
(5) Prochlorperazine (Compazine) 10 mg stat. and every 3-4 hours p.r.n. for nausea IM

Laboratory Results

Serum sodium	144 mEq/L
Serum potassium	4.2 mEq/L
Serum chloride	104 mEq/L
Carbon dioxide	23 mEq/L

Blood urea nitrogen	20 mg/100 ml
Serum glucose	178 mg/100 ml
Hemoglobin	17.9 gm/100 ml
Hematocrit	54.6%
Urine specific gravity	1.038

10:15 A.M. Prochlorperazine 10 mg was given IM.

2:00 P.M. Meperidine 50 mg with promethazine 25 mg was given IM for pain. Mr. Chang stated that he no longer was nauseated. He dozed most of the afternoon and stated he was very drowsy.

Medical Orders

(1) Intravenous fluids as follows:
 Left ankle — 2000 ml 5% glucose in water
 Add potassium chloride 20 mEq and vitamin B & C (Folbesyn) one ampule to first bottle of 5% glucose in water
 CVP line — 2000 ml lactated Ringer's solution
 Salt poor albumin 100 ml IV stat.
 Regulate IV's to total 150-200 ml/hour
(2) Surgical liquid diet in A.M.
(3) Aluminum hydroxide and magnesium trisilicate gel (Gelusil) 30 ml q.i.d. (to start in A.M.)

On examination, Mr. Chang's chest was clear to auscultation and percussion; abdomen soft; bowel sounds present.

Study Questions

32. Why was morphine discontinued at 10:00 A.M. on the second hospital day?

33. What is the purpose of administration of meperidine with promethazine?

34. What clinical observations would indicate that IM administration of the narcotic analgesic is no longer dangerous?

35. What is the pharmacological action of prochlorperazine? Discuss the nursing assessment for side and adverse effects.

36. What evidence is there that prochlorperazine may have been effective?

37. What is the probable explanation for Mr. Chang's drowsiness in the afternoon of the second hospital day?

38. Why is potassium chloride being added to the intravenous infusion even though the serum potassium was within normal range?

39. What roles do vitamins B and C play in metabolism? Besides the fact that Mr. Chang is NPO, what other reason is there for vitamin B and C administration to the burn patient?

40. What is the rationale for Gelusil administration to Mr. Chang?

Laboratory Results (4:00 P.M.)

Serum osmolality 310 mOs/kg

4:00 P.M. Acetaminophen 600 mg suppository was administered and both intravenous infusions were adjusted to run at 100 ml/hour. Prior to 4:00 P.M. the intravenous infusions ran at 65 and 125 ml/hour. Physician was notified about output below 50 ml.

5:00 P.M. Urine output and vital signs remained adequate throughout the rest of the second day.

11:45 P.M. 24-Hour Intake and Output
Intake: 4640 ml IV Output: 1250 ml

FLOW SHEET — SECOND HOSPITAL DAY

Time	Temp	Pulse	Resp	BP	CVP	IV # 1	IV # 2	Output
1 A.M.		112	22	114/74	7.0	65 ml	125 ml	50 ml
2 A.M.	99.6	110	24	110/68	7.0	65 ml	125 ml	55 ml
3 A.M.		112	22	108/58	6.5	65 ml	125 ml	55 ml
4 A.M.	99.8	112	22	112/72	7.0	65 ml	125 ml	50 ml
5 A.M.		114	24	112/72	7.0	65 ml	125 ml	55 ml
6 A.M.	100	116	24	110/60	7.0	65 ml	125 ml	50 ml
7 A.M.		118	24	114/58	7.0	65 ml	125 ml	50 ml
8 A.M.	101.6	128	28	112/80	7.0	65 ml	125 ml	55 ml
9 A.M.	100	116	24	110/60	7.0	65 ml	125 ml	50 ml
10 A.M.	100	118	24	118/72	7.0	65 ml	125 ml	55 ml
11 A.M.	100	116	24	114/64		65 ml	125 ml	60 ml
12 P.M.	100.2	120	24	110/60	7.0	65 ml	125 ml	50 ml
1 P.M.	100	118	24	110/60		65 ml	125 ml	50 ml
2 P.M.	100.4	120	24	112/72		65 ml	125 ml	50 ml
3 P.M.	100.6	120	24	114/60		65 ml	125 ml	50 ml
4 P.M.	101	124	24	108/50	6.0	65 ml	125 ml	35 ml
5 P.M.	99.8	106	22	110/60	6.5	100 ml	100 ml	50 ml
6 P.M.	99.8	108	24	110/58		100 ml	100 ml	60 ml
7 P.M.		110	24	112/72		100 ml	100 ml	50 ml
8 P.M.	99.8	112	24	108/60	6.5	100 ml	100 ml	55 ml
9 P.M.		114	24	110/80		100 ml	100 ml	55 ml
10 P.M.	99.6	110	22	110/60		100 ml	100 ml	50 ml
11 P.M.		110	24	112/72		100 ml	100 ml	55 ml
12 A.M.	99.6	112	22	110/60	7.0	100 ml	110 ml	50 ml

Study Questions

41. What is the relationship of acetaminophen administered to Mr. Chang's current metabolic state?

42. What are the possible reasons for the temperature elevation?

43. Discuss the rationale for decreasing total fluids administered on the second hospital day.

44. Why is salt-poor albumin ordered again?

45. Discuss the interpretation of data available to the nurse in her decision to increase the IV flow rate at 4:00 P.M. What follow-up should the nurse make to evaluate the patient's physiological response to this action?

Third Hospital Day

Laboratory Results (12:00 A.M.)

Serum osmolality	304 mOs/kg

8:00 A.M. Mr. Chang refused liquids at breakfast and complained of abdominal discomfort. His abdomen appeared slightly distended and was tympanic to percussion.

Medical Orders

(1) Intravenous fluids as follows:
 2000 ml 5% glucose in water, add one ampule vitamin B and C to first bottle of glucose in water
 2000 ml lactated Ringer's solution
(2) Discontinue serum osmolalities
(3) Soap suds enema now
(4) Wound cultures daily

9:00 A.M. The enema was given and Mr. Chang expelled some flatus and a moderate amount of formed brown stool. He seemed less distended and more comfortable. CVP measurements and vital signs were within normal limits with the exception of a temperature of 100.6° F. at noon and 101° F. at 4:00 P.M. An acetaminophen suppository 600 mg was administered with resulting reduction in temperature.

Laboratory Results (10:00 A.M.)

Serum sodium	139 mEq/L
Serum potassium	3.4 mEq/L
Serum chloride	99 mEq/L
Carbon dioxide	27 mEq/L
Blood urea nitrogen	18 mg/100 ml
Serum glucose	225 mg/100 ml

Hemoglobin	16.9 gm/100 ml
Hematocrit	48.5%
Urine specific gravity	1.028

Mr. Chang experienced no respiratory distress and seemed fairly comfortable with the exception of the times silver sulfadiazine cream was reapplied to his burns. His output averaged between 50 and 60 ml per hour.

Fourth Hospital Day

Medical Orders

(1) Intravenous fluids as follows:
    2000 ml 5% glucose in water, add one ampule vitamin B and C to first bottle of glucose in water
    2000 ml lactated Ringer's solution
    Regulate IV's to run at 150 ml/hour
(2) Discontinue aluminum hydroxide and magnesium trisilicate gel (Gelusil)
(3) Calcium carbonate and glycine (Titralac) 2 tablets q.i.d.
(4) Discontinue CVP measurements but do not discontinue CVP line
(5) Discontinue daily electrolytes
(6) Discontinue cutdown in left ankle
(7) Vital signs every 4 hours
(8) Transfer to private room on surgical ward
(9) Maintain reverse isolation

Mr. Chang was transferred from the intensive care unit to a surgical unit. He was placed on a regular bed. He was given meperidine and promethazine after he was transferred because the move seemed to cause much discomfort for him. He received acetaminophen suppositories 600 mg three times on the fourth hospital day for temperature elevations. He was able to tolerate the liquid diet well.

Laboratory Results

Serum sodium	139 mEq/L
Serum potassium	3.4 mEq/L
Serum chloride	101 mEq/L
Carbon dioxide	38 mEq/L
Blood urea nitrogen	20 mg/100 ml
Serum glucose	168 mg/100 ml
Hemoglobin	16.4 gm/100 ml
Hematocrit	47%

24-Hour Intake and Output

Intake:	4430 ml IV	Output:	3350 ml
	880 ml p.o.		

Study Questions

46. Describe the difference in composition of Gelusil and Titralac. What are the advantages and disadvantages of each?

47. What is the action of Titralac? What instructions should the nurse give Mr. Chang when administering Titralac tablets?

48. What ion, contained in Titralac, is frequently deficient in the burn patient? Discuss how this deficiency occurs.

Fifth Hospital Day

Medical Orders (9:00 A.M.)

(1) Whirlpool daily with pHisoHEX (physical therapy)
(2) Up in chair
(3) Soft diet
(4) Intravenous fluids as follows:
2000 ml 5% glucose in water, add one ampule vitamin B and C to first bottle of glucose in water
2000 ml lactated Ringer's solution
Regulate IV's to run at 125 ml/hour
(5) Serum electrolytes in A.M.

Mr. Chang's burns of his extremities were edematous and oozing. He continued to have elevated temperatures between 100° and 101.2° F. for which he received acetaminophen suppositories.

Laboratory Results

Wound culture	no growth

24-Hour Intake and Output

Intake:	3430 ml IV	Output:	4775 ml
	2490 ml p.o.		

Sixth Hospital Day

Medical Orders

(1) Intravenous fluids as follows:
1000 ml 5% glucose in water, add one ampule vitamin B and C to this bottle only
3000 ml lactated Ringer's solution
Regulate IV's to run at 125 ml/hour
(2) Reduce aqueous penicillin to 500,000 units every 8 hours per metriset

Laboratory Results

Serum sodium	139 mEq/L
Serum potassium	2.8 mEq/L
Serum chloride	94 mEq/L
Carbon dioxide	32 mEq/L
Blood urea nitrogen	4 mg/100 ml
Serum glucose	117 mg/100 ml
Hemoglobin	13.5 gm/100 ml
Hematocrit	40.1%
Urine specific gravity	1.009
Wound culture	no growth

Mr. Chang was able to ambulate to the chair. He had difficulty sitting and preferred to walk or stand. He complained of abdominal distention — a full feeling — and did not seem to have much appetite. He stated that he felt very tired and weaker than yesterday but did not require pain medication.

24-Hour Intake and Output

Intake:	3850 ml IV	Output:	5070 ml
	2320 ml p.o.		

Seventh Hospital Day

Medical Orders

(1) Ambulate
(2) High protein, high carbohydrate, 2000 Calorie diet
(3) Discontinue intravenous fluids
(4) Discontinue Foley catheter
(5) Sulfamethoxazole and phenazopyridine (AzoGantanol) 2 tablets stat., then 2 tablets b.i.d.
(6) Potassium chloride (K-Lor) 20 mEq p.o. t.i.d. p.c.
(7) Discontinue meperidine hydrochloride (Demerol), and promethazine (Phenergan)
(8) Acetaminophen with 30 mg codeine phosphate (Tylenol # 3) every 4-6 hours p.r.n. for pain p.o.
(9) Flurazepam hydrochloride (Dalmane) 30 mg h.s. p.r.n.
(10) Weigh patient today

Mr. Chang's Foley catheter was removed at noon, and his intravenous infusion was discontinued at 2:00 P.M. He was able to void 200 to 600 ml at a time. His burn wounds continued to ooze serous fluid. His weight was 152 pounds.

Laboratory Results

Wound culture	no growth

24-Hour Intake and Output

Intake:	3320 ml IV	Output:	5000 ml
	2360 ml p.o.		

Eighth to Fourteenth Hospital Days

Mr. Chang continued to improve and became very eager to leave the hospital. He wanted to know how long he would need to remain confined to his hospital room. He began to complain of pain more frequently in the evening and had difficulty sleeping. His wound cultures continued to show no growth. His appetite was excellent and he gained 4 pounds prior to discharge 14 days after he sustained his burns. He was discharged with dressings to his hands and thighs. He was instructed to dress his hand and thigh wounds following application of silver sulfadiazine cream and to continue application of silver sulfadiazine to other open burn areas.

Study Questions

49. Considering the change in urinary output on the fourth hospital day, what precautions are necessary in intravenous fluid administration? Why?

50. Relate the increased lactated Ringer's solution order to the burn wound healing process, the laboratory test values, and body fluid mechanisms.

51. What is the purpose for the addition of pHisoHEX to the whirlpool bath? What purpose does the whirlpool serve in relation to drug therapy?

52. Why is acetaminophen preferred over aspirin for this patient?

53. Discuss the reason for the potassium chloride order on the seventh hospital day.

54. Describe other nursing interventions which might decrease the need for the potassium chloride order.

55. What are the expected outcomes of potassium chloride therapy which may be observed by the nurse?

56. What is the action of sulfamethoxazole and phenazopyridine? Why was it ordered for Mr. Chang on the seventh hospital day? What patient teaching is needed regarding this drug?

57. Relate the changes in pain medication order to the change in Mr. Chang's pain behavior. What additional nursing interventions are indicated at this time relative to Mr. Chang's complaints regarding pain?

58. Describe the action of flurazepam and the reason it was ordered on the seventh hospital day for Mr. Chang. Discuss the nurse's evaluation for the administration of this p.r.n. medication.

59. Why wasn't an iron compound ordered for Mr. Chang? At what point in time following the burn would an anemia be evident? What other therapy is often pre-

scribed related to postburn anemia?

60. What is the significance of the daily wound culture reports?

61. Describe discharge teaching needed to continue effective burn wound management.

REFERENCES

Artz, C. P., and Moncrief, J. A.: The Treatment of Burns, ed. 3. W. B. Saunders Co., Philadelphia, 1974.

Baxter, C., Marvin, J., and Curreri, P. W.: Fluid and electrolyte therapy in burn shock. Heart Lung, 2:707-713, 1973.

Hunt, J., et al.: Burn wound management. Heart Lung, 2:690-695, 1973.

Jacoby, F.: Nursing Care of the Patient with Burns. C. V. Mosby Co., St. Louis, 1972.

Jelenko, C.: Systemic response to burn injury: a survey of some current concepts. J. Trauma 10:877-883, 1970.

Metheny, N., and Snively, Jr., W. D.: Nurses' Handbook of Fluid Balance, ed. 2. J.B. Lippincott Co., Philadelphia, 1974.

20

THE PATIENT WITH DIABETES MELLITUS

TEXTBOOKS SUGGESTED FOR THIS STUDY

Asperheim, M. K., and Eisenhauer, L. A.: The Pharmacologic Basis of Patient Care, ed. 2. W. B. Saunders Co., Philadelphia, 1973, Chapters 6, 9, and 15.

Bergersen, B.: Pharmacology in Nursing, ed. 13. C. V. Mosby Co., St. Louis, 1976, Chapter 25.

Brunner, L. S., and Suddarth, D.: Textbook of Medical Surgical Nursing, ed. 3. J.B. Lippincott Co., Philadelphia, 1975, Chapter 32.

Goodman, L., and Gilman, A. (eds.): The Pharmacological Basis of Therapeutics, ed. 5. Macmillan Co., New York, 1975, Chapter 71.

Luckmann, J., and Sorensen, K.: Medical-Surgical Nursing — A Psychophysiologic Approach. W. B. Saunders Co., Philadelphia, 1974, Chapter 95.

Rodman, M. J., and Smith, D.: Clinical Pharmacology in Nursing. J. B. Lippincott Co., Philadelphia, 1974, Chapter 39.

Shafer, K. N., et al.: Medical Surgical Nursing, ed. 6. C. V. Mosby Co., St. Louis, 1975, Chapter 27.

PAST MEDICAL HISTORY

Barbara Lester is a 16-year-old high school student with a history of relatively good health. During the last six months, a growth spurt increased her height to 66 inches. Despite an increased appetite and food intake, Barbara lost 10 pounds over the last two months, resulting in a weight of 102 pounds.

When Barbara came home from school one Friday, she appeared ill. She complained of fatigue and nausea, refused dinner, and went straight to bed. The next morning Barbara woke up nauseated and began vomiting and having diarrhea. She was very weak and drowsy and stumbled going to and from the bathroom.

Nausea, vomiting, and diarrhea continued during the morning and Barbara became increasingly drowsy. Her parents called the family doctor who said that he would meet them at the local hospital emergency room as soon as they could get there.

PRESENT HOSPITAL ADMISSION

First Hospital Day

Barbara was admitted to the emergency room in a semicomatose state at 1:00 P.M.

Her vital signs were temperature 99.8° F. (rectally), blood pressure 84/40, pulse 108, and respirations 36. Breath odor was fruity, and her abdomen appeared somewhat distended. She vomited a small amount of russet liquid. The nurse noted that her lips and mouth were dry and she had a dry furry tongue. Her skin was flushed and her extremities were cool and dry.

Medical Orders (1:03 P.M.)

(1) Blood glucose stat.
(2) Plasma ketone stat.
(3) Insert indwelling catheter
(4) Check urine stat. for glucose (Clinitest) and acetone (Ketostix)
(5) Start 1000 ml normal saline
(6) Hourly intake and output

The physician drew the blood specimen and started the intravenous infusion as the nurse inserted the indwelling catheter and checked the first specimen of concentrated urine. Urine sugar was 4+ and ketone large. The rest of the urine specimen was sent to the laboratory for further analysis. Part of the blood specimen was checked immediately in the emergency room for glucose and acetone using a paper reagent strip (Dextrostix and Acetest). Both tests were strongly positive.

Medical Orders

(1) U-100 Regular Insulin (beef-pork) 50 units by intravenous bolus stat.
(2) Infuse present 1000 ml normal saline intravenously over the next 1½ hours; then give 1000 ml normal saline over the following 3½ hours
(3) Vital signs every 30 minutes until stable, then every hour
(4) Additional laboratory tests stat.
    Complete blood count and differential
    Hemoglobin
    Hematocrit
    Serum sodium, chloride, potassium, and carbon dioxide
    Blood pH and repeat every hour
(5) Blood glucose every hour
(6) Plasma ketone every hour
(7) Cardiac monitor
(8) Hourly intake and output
(9) Hourly urines for sugar (Clinitest) and acetone (Ketostix)
(10) Insert nasogastric tube and connect to low gumco suction

1:08 P.M. The intravenous insulin was administered and the hourly urine collections were initiated.

1:10 P.M. The initial laboratory report confirmed a 4+ plasma ketone level and revealed a blood glucose level of 588 mg/100 ml. A medical diagnosis of metabolic ketoacidosis and diabetes mellitus was made. Barbara was transferred to the Intensive Care Unit.

1:30 P.M. Barbara continued to be difficult to arouse. Vomiting stopped when the nasogastric tube was inserted. Her deep tendon reflexes were normal. Vital signs were blood pressure 90/48, pulse 108, and respirations 32 with a continued fruity odor.

Laboratory Results

Red blood count		5.5 million per cu mm
Hemoglobin		14 gm/100 ml
Hematocrit		52%
White blood count:		14,000 per cu mm
(differential)		
Polys	82%	
Eosinophils	3%	
Lymphocytes	15%	
Serum sodium		139 mEq/L
Serum potassium		3.7 mEq/L
Serum chloride		100 mEq/L
Blood pH		7.2
Plasma ketone		4+

2:00 P.M. Barbara continued to be difficult to arouse. Her urine output for the hour since admission was 25 ml, and the 2:00 P.M. urine check showed 4+ sugar and a large amount of ketone. Intravenous intake during the first hour was 600 ml. Her vital signs were blood pressure 100/48, pulse 92, and respirations 32. The 2:00 P.M. blood glucose level was 400 mg/100 ml, plasma ketone 3+, and blood pH 7.25.

Medical Orders

(1) U-100 Regular Insulin (beef-pork) 25 units by intravenous bolus stat.
(2) U-100 Regular Insulin (beef-pork) 25 units by s.c. stat.
(3) Repeat serum potassium hourly

Study Questions

1. What is the action of Regular Insulin and why was it administered to Barbara?

2. Discuss the action of insulin as it is related to the metabolic changes present in Barbara at the time of her admission. Include results of Barbara's laboratory tests.

3. Why was the intravenous route selected for the administration of the insulin? Discuss how the insulin should be prepared and administered to Barbara.

4. Compare Regular Insulin with other types of insulin in relation to administration during ketoacidosis. Include routes of administration as well as time, peak, and duration of action following administration.

5. Compare the intravenous, intramuscular, and subcutaneous methods for administration of insulin. Which methods are used for emergency situations? Why was the method of administration of Regular Insulin changed from intravenous push only at

1:10 P.M. to intravenous push and subcutaneous at 2:00 P.M.?

6. Discuss the use of continuous low-dose infusion of insulin and compare this method with the method used to treat Barbara's ketoacidosis. How would nursing responsibilities differ in the implementation of each method?

7. What electrolytes are provided in the intravenous fluids being administered to Barbara? Relate the laboratory test results to the fluids ordered.

8. Why did the physician order rapid infusion of the intravenous infusion?

9. What should be included in Barbara's nursing assessment to determine the effectiveness of the insulin administration? What signs and symptoms would indicate a positive response? How would adverse effects be recognized?

10. Barbara was ill for a number of hours before coming to the emergency room. Discuss why stat. laboratory tests, intravenous fluids, and insulin are necessary for her treatment.

11. Evaluate Barbara's blood pH level in view of the acid-base imbalance usual in diabetic ketoacidosis. What relationship is there between the blood pH level and the use of normal saline for intravenous infusion?

12. Sodium bicarbonate is sometimes administered for patients with ketoacidosis. Discuss reasons why the physician did not order it for Barbara when the blood pH level was reported.

2:30 P.M. While the nurse was checking her vital signs, Barbara began to move around a bit and was more easily aroused. She said her mouth was dry and she was very thirsty. Vital signs were blood pressure 104/68, pulse 92, and respirations 28. Urinary output began to increase and the intravenous infusion was running well. Barbara's chest was clear, and her abdomen was soft. A small amount of brown drainage was present in the nasogastric suction bottle.

Laboratory Results (3:00 P.M.)

Blood glucose	300 mg/100 ml
Plasma ketone	2+
Blood pH	7.3
Serum potassium	3.5 mEq/L
Urine glucose	4+
Urine ketone	moderate

Medical Orders

U-100 Regular Insulin (beef-pork) 25 units by s.c. now.

Barbara's urinary output continued to improve, her second hour of urinary output totaled 40 ml and contained 4+ sugar and moderate ketone. Intravenous intake during the second hour was 540 ml. Barbara was more awake and began to move about more in bed. Her vital signs were blood pressure 104/68, pulse 90, and respirations 28. Regular Insulin 25 units was administered by s.c. injection.

3:30 P.M. Barbara's vital signs were blood pressure 106/68, pulse 90, and respirations 28.

Laboratory Results (4:00 P.M.)

Blood glucose	250 mg/100 ml
Plasma ketone	1+
Serum potassium	3.4 mEq/L
Blood pH	7.3
Urine glucose	4+
Urine ketone	moderate

Medical Orders

(1) U-100 Regular Insulin (beef-pork) 20 units s.c. now
(2) Add 40 mEq potassium chloride to the present intravenous bottle and administer over the next 2 hours

Barbara's vital signs were temperature 98.8° F., blood pressure 106/68, pulse 90, and respirations 26. Urine output from 3:00 P.M. to 4:00 P.M. was 40 ml and intravenous intake 290 ml. The nurse administered the s.c. insulin and added the potassium chloride to the intravenous infusion. Barbara was encouraged to deep breathe and cough. Although still drowsy, Barbara was able to talk with the nurse. She said that she had not been feeling well lately but thought it was just the flu. She wanted to know what was in the bottle of intravenous fluid and why she had been receiving injections. She continued to complain of thirst. There was no additional drainage in the nasogastric suction bottle, and Barbara's abdomen appeared to be flat.

Study Questions

13. Discuss further indications of the effects of insulin on Barbara's signs and symptoms. Include laboratory results as well as Barbara's quantitative and qualitative responses.

14. What evidence points to the need for the order for potassium chloride to be added to the intravenous infusion?

15. How should the potassium chloride be prepared and administered to Barbara?

16. What precautions should the nurse take in administering potassium chloride to Barbara? What relationships are there between the administration of potassium chloride and Barbara's urinary output? What changes would point to the need for decreasing the administration rate of potassium chloride and for notifying the physician?

17. Discuss the relationship between the administration of insulin to Barbara and the administration of potassium chloride.

18. Discuss what responses would be appropriate to Barbara's questions about the content of the intravenous fluids and the injections.

<u>Laboratory Results</u> (5:00 P.M.)

Blood glucose	220 mg/100 ml
Plasma ketone	1+
Serum potassium	3.5 mEq/L
Blood pH	7.3
Urine glucose	4+
Urine ketone	moderate

<u>Medical Orders</u>

(1) U-100 Regular Insulin (beef-pork) 20 units s.c. now
(2) Clamp off nasogastric tube

Barbara's vital signs were blood pressure 104/68, pulse 90, and respirations 24. Intake and output for the previous hour totaled urinary output 50 ml and intravenous intake 280 ml. The nurse clamped off the nasogastric tube and noted that Barbara's abdomen had remained soft. Chest sounds were normal.

<u>Laboratory Results</u> (6:00 P.M.)

Blood glucose	190 mg/100 ml
Plasma ketone	1+
Serum potassium	3.5 mEq/L
Blood pH	7.35
Urine glucose	3+
Urine ketone	small

<u>Medical Orders</u>

(1) U-100 Regular Insulin (beef-pork) 15 units s.c. now
(2) Remove nasogastric tube and begin sips of broth and juices not to exceed 100 ml/hour
(3) Follow present intravenous infusion with 1000 ml 5% glucose in 0.45% sodium chloride solution with 40 mEq potassium chloride. Infuse at 150 ml/hour
(4) Remove the urinary catheter

Barbara's vital signs were blood pressure 106/60, pulse 88, and respirations 22. Intake and output for the previous hour totaled urinary output 60 ml and intravenous intake 290 ml. Barbara was glad to have the nasogastric tube removed and had a few sips of beef broth. The nurse attached the next intravenous bottle and removed the urinary catheter.

<u>Laboratory Results</u> (7:00 P.M.)

Blood glucose	185 mg/100 ml

Plasma ketone	1+
Serum potassium	3.7 mEq/L
Blood pH	7.35
Urine glucose	2+
Urine ketone	small

Medical Orders

U-100 Regular Insulin (beef-pork) 15 units s.c. now

Barbara's vital signs were blood pressure 106/60, pulse 86, and respirations 22. Barbara got up to the bathroom with the nurse's assistance and voided 70 ml of clear urine. Intake over the previous hour included 150 ml of intravenous fluid and sips of broth and juice totaling 50 ml. Barbara said that her mouth felt a little less dry, and she was able to tolerate small sips of broth and fruit juice.

Study Questions

19. Discuss the relationship between the continued changes in laboratory results and the orders for insulin administration.

20. What indications point to the need for intravenous potassium chloride? What additional sources of potassium chloride have been started?

21. What indications are present for the change of intravenous infusion solutions from normal saline to 5% glucose in 0.45% sodium chloride solution? Why is glucose administered when the blood glucose level is elevated?

22. Identify the sites used for the administration of s.c. insulin. What methods should be used to plan for rotation of these sites in the administration of Barbara's insulin? What methods can be used to insure site rotation when different nurses on different shifts administer s.c. insulin to the same patient?

23. Explain how the method of administration of insulin can enhance its effectiveness.

24. What factors increase insulin requirements? What factors decrease insulin requirements?

Laboratory Results (8:00 P.M.)

Blood glucose	220 mg/100 ml
Plasma ketone	negative
Serum potassium	3.7 mEq/L
Blood pH	7.35
Urine glucose	2+
Urine ketone	negative

Medical Orders

(1) Change the following hourly laboratory tests to every 4 hours:
  Blood glucose
  Plasma ketone
  Serum potassium
(2) Change urine sugar and acetone testing to every 4 hours
(3) Repeat the following in the A.M.:
  Complete blood count and differential
  Serum sodium, chloride, potassium, and carbon dioxide
  Blood pH
(4) Continue administration of 5% glucose in 0.45% sodium chloride solution with 40 mEq potassium chloride to each 1000 ml of fluid at 150 ml/hour
(5) U-100 Regular Insulin (beef-pork) 20 units s.c. now
(6) Administer U-100 Regular Insulin at 12:00 A.M. and 4:00 A.M. according to the following scale:

Blood glucose level	Insulin Administration
Below 200 mg/100 ml	Omit Regular Insulin
200-250 mg/100 ml	5 units Regular Insulin s.c.
250-350 mg/100 ml	10 units Regular Insulin s.c.
Above 350 mg/100 ml	15 units Regular Insulin s.c.

(7) Vital signs every 4 hours

Barbara's vital signs were temperature 99.0° F., blood pressure 108/68, pulse 88, and respirations 24. The intake from 7:00 P.M. to 8:00 P.M. was 150 ml intravenous and 50 ml of juice; the output was 65 ml. The nurse administered the Regular Insulin s.c. and offered Barbara a glass of juice. Barbara drank the juice and said that she felt really worn out, and was glad that the nurse would not be in to check her vital signs quite as often during the night. Barbara settled down and fell asleep.

Laboratory Results (12:00 A.M.)

Blood glucose	180 mg/100 ml
Plasma ketone	negative
Serum potassium	3.6 mEq/L
Blood pH	7.35
Urine glucose	2+
Urine ketone	negative

Barbara's vital signs were temperature 98.2° F., blood pressure 108/68, pulse 88, and respirations 24. Barbara was asleep when the nurse aroused her and fell asleep shortly thereafter. Total intake and output since admission were as follows:

Intake: 2900 ml intravenous
  250 ml oral

Output: 530 ml urine

Laboratory Results (4:00 A.M.)

Blood glucose	208 mg/100 ml
Plasma Ketone	negative
Serum potassium	3.7 mEq/L
Blood pH	7.35
Urine glucose	3+
Urine ketone	negative

Barbara continued to sleep following the midnight vital signs but was easily aroused at 4:00 A.M. Her vital signs were temperature 98.0° F., blood pressure 104/60, pulse 72, and respirations 20. The nurse administered 5 units of Regular Insulin s.c. Barbara's chest was clear, her abdomen remained soft, and she stated that she felt much less thirsty. Barbara fell back asleep after taking some sips of a cup of beef broth.

Study Questions

25. Discuss the reasons for the change at 8:00 P.M. from hourly to every 4 hour laboratory observations of Barbara. Include subjective as well as objective changes in Barbara's status.

26. Relate the changes in serum potassium level to the need for continued administration of intravenous potassium chloride. How would the nurse evaluate the effectiveness of this medication? What side effects should be anticipated in evaluating Barbara's reaction to the medication?

27. Discuss the implementation of the order at 8:00 P.M. which includes a variety of insulin dosages dependent on the blood glucose levels. What are the legal implications for this kind of a medication order? Compare the use and accuracy of blood glucose and urine sugar in the implementation of this kind of an order.

28. Why was there no insulin administered at 12:00 A.M.?

29. Discuss the intake and output totals observed at 12:00 A.M. and relate the results to the need for administration of intravenous fluids and insulin. In light of the totals, the nurse should be evaluating Barbara for what complications? What would this evaluation include and how is it carried out?

30. What was the basis for administration of 5 units of U-100 Regular Insulin at 4:00 A.M.?

Second Hospital Day

Laboratory Results (7:00 A.M.)

Blood glucose	180 mg/100 ml
Plasma ketone	negative
Serum potassium	3.7 mEq/L
Blood pH	7.35
Urine glucose	2+
Urine ketone	negative

Barbara awoke easily for vital signs which were temperature 97.8° F., blood pressure 104/68, pulse 72, and respirations 18. She was hungry and asked the nurse if she could have something besides juice and broth for breakfast. The nurse called the physician to report the 7:00 A.M. blood glucose and asked him about giving Barbara a diet.

Medical Orders

(1) Start 2000 Calorie diabetic diet this A.M.
(2) 15 units of U-100 NPH Insulin (beef-pork) s.c. every A.M.
(3) Serial blood glucose levels for 2 days (fasting, 11:00 A.M., 3:00 P.M., and 9:00 P.M.)
(4) 24-hour urine for glucose and protein
(5) 24-hour urine for creatinine clearance
(6) 24-hour urine for 17-ketosteroids and 17-hydroxycorticoids
(7) Blood urea nitrogen, total protein, SGOT, prothrombin time, bilirubin, lipids, and PBI
(8) Chest x-ray
(9) Urine sugar and acetone testing q.i.d. a.c. and h.s.
(10) Continue to administer U-100 Regular Insulin (beef-pork) according to the following scale:

Blood glucose level	Insulin Administration
Below 200 mg/100 ml	Omit Regular Insulin
200-250 mg/100 ml	5 units Regular Insulin s.c.
250-350 mg/100 ml	10 units Regular Insulin s.c.
Above 350 mg/100 ml	15 units Regular Insulin s.c.

(11) Transfer to regular medical unit

The nurse administered the 15 units of U-100 NPH Insulin to Barbara. She ate all of her breakfast and was then transferred to the regular medical unit. Her vital signs continued to be stable and her intravenous infusions were discontinued. She was able to get up and move around more and said she felt much better but still weak and shaky. Lunch and dinner were taken well.

Laboratory Results — Second Hospital Day

Time	Blood Glucose	Urine Sugar	Urine Ketone
11:00 A.M.	150 mg/100 ml	negative	negative
3:00 P.M.	140 mg/100 ml	negative	negative
9:00 P.M.	170 mg/100 ml	negative	negative

Third to Fifth Hospital Days

Barbara continued to do well and began learning about insulin injections, urine testing, and diabetes mellitus in general. Her dosage of U-100 NPH Insulin was gradually increased to 35 units each A.M. and the blood glucose levels gradually came down to between 100 mg/100 ml and 150 mg/100 ml for fasting specimens. Barbara complained of some swelling of her legs and feet, and the nurse told her that it was temporary and would probably be gone in a few days. She encouraged her to report further changes. Blood glucose levels were changed from four times a day to two times a day (fasting and at 3:00 P.M.)

Study Questions

31. Why did the nurse call the physician at 7:00 A.M. to report the blood glucose level?

32. What is the difference between Regular Insulin and NPH Insulin? Include routes of administration; onset, peak, and duration of action; and side effects in the discussion.

33. U-100 NPH Insulin has been ordered for Barbara. Compare it to U-40 and U-80. Include advantages, disadvantages, and equipment needed for the administration of each kind of insulin.

34. Why has the physician continued to order Regular Insulin according to blood glucose levels, in addition to starting the administration of NPH Insulin for Barbara?

35. Identify the aspects of insulin administration that should be included in teaching Barbara to administer her own insulin. How should the nurse determine whether Barbara is ready to learn about insulin administration? How would the nurse evaluate Barbara's ability in relation to insulin administration? Include injection technique, care of the equipment, and knowledge of the medication in the discussion.

36. Relate Barbara's complaint of leg and feet swelling to the administration of NPH Insulin. Is the nurse's comment justified? What additional reactions should the nurse be alert to, how common are their occurrences, and what interventions would be appropriate?

37. At what time should the nurse be looking for insulin reactions to occur following the initiation of NPH Insulin for Barbara?

38. How does the order for Barbara's diabetic diet relate to the dosage of insulin ordered?

39. What adjustments are possible in relation to the distribution of the diet throughout the day to cover the various properties of NPH Insulin?

Fifth Hospital Day

2:00 P.M. The nurse arrived in Barbara's room for the scheduled afternoon teaching session, and found Barbara irritable and somewhat confused. She was lethargic and unable to carry out an intelligent conversation. The nurse brought Barbara a glass of orange juice, called the physician, obtained a stat. blood glucose level, and tested Barbara's urine for sugar and acetone. The blood glucose level was 60 mg/100 ml and the urine negative for both sugar and acetone. Two hours later a repeat blood glucose showed 100 mg/100 ml, and Barbara said she felt normal again. The daily order for U-100 Regular Insulin was changed to 25 units every A.M.

Study Questions

40. Identify the cause of the symptoms Barbara experienced during the afternoon of the fifth hospital day. What are the reasons for the nursing actions instituted? Can additional episodes be avoided?

41. What are the damaging effects of a hypoglycemic attack such as Barbara experienced? Identify body functions that can be damaged or changed by such an event.

Sixth through Tenth Hospital Days

Barbara adjusted to the revised insulin dosage, and made rapid progress in the diabetic teaching program. She was discharged from the hospital on the tenth hospital day, with a referral to the Visiting Nurse Association.

Study Questions

42. During the course of learning to give her own injections, Barbara asked the nurse whether she could take pills instead of injections for her diabetes. What would be an appropriate response to this question?

43. Compare the use, advantages, and disadvantages of oral hypoglycemics with insulin, and discuss why insulin is used to treat Barbara's disease.

44. What other methods should Barbara be taught to institute when she begins to feel a hypoglycemic attack?

45. Discuss the physiological and psychosocial factors that may influence Barbara's ability to adjust to the diagnosis of diabetes mellitus and insulin administration.

46. Discuss the factors that both increase and decrease the body's requirements for insulin.

47. Two days before discharge, Barbara told the nurse that she was going to follow the doctor's orders carefully and take her insulin every day because she wanted to be cured as soon as possible. What should the nurse include in her assessment of Barbara to develop a realistic teaching plan?

48. Develop a teaching plan for Barbara. Include proper storage of her medication, time of administration, and a discussion of insulin reactions in your answer.

49. What should the nurse say to Barbara in response to her statement about wanting to be cured?

REFERENCES

Carozza, V.: Diabetic out of control — nursing grand rounds. Nursing '73, 3:11-15, 1973.

Diabetes Mellitus, ed. 7. Lilly Research Laboratories, Indianapolis, 1973.

Dolger, H., and Seeman, B.: The diabetic adolescent. In How to Live With Diabetes.

Pyramid Books, New York, 1965, pp. 138-149.
Engle, V.: Diabetic teaching — how to win your patient's cooperation in his care. Nursing '75, 5:17-24, 1975.
Giolot, D. H., and McKinney, N. P.: Administering parenteral drugs. Am. J. Nurs., 75:788-793, 1975
Grancio, S. D.: Nursing care of the adult diabetic patient. Nurs. Clin. N. Am., 8: 605-615, 1973.
Guthrie, D., and Guthrie, R.: Diabetes in adolescence. Am. J. Nurs., 75:1740-1744, 1975.
Kitabchi, A. E., Ayyagari, V., and Guerra, S.: The efficacy of low-dose versus conventional therapy of insulin for treatment of diabetic ketoacidosis. Ann. Intern. Med., 84:633-638, 1976.
Newmark, S. R., Himathongkam, T., and Shane, J. M.: Hyperglycemic and hypoglycemic crises. J.A.M.A. 231:185-187, 1975.
Shumann, D.: Assessing the diabetic. Nursing '76, 6:62-67, 1976.
Smith, S. E.: Antidiabetic drugs. Nurs. Times, 71:1744-1745, 1975.